DITCH THE DIET

Conquer Your Cravings, Accelerate Your Fat Loss
and Boost Your Energy Levels

Tyson Brown

Let's Tell Your Story
London

COPYRIGHT

DISCLAIMER

The opinions and suggestions reflect the research and ideas of the author and aren't intended to substitute for services by a medical professional. All content here is for informational purposes only and should not be taken as medical advice. The author assumes no responsibility for any adverse effects resulting from information in this book.

Tyson's disclaimer:

Treat this book as a guide – as useful information that will help you make a sound judgement on improving your health and well-being.

Always consult a doctor or specialist before doing before embarking on a new diet, lifestyle or fitness regime.

Affiliate Discloser:

Some of the recommendations provided in the book link to websites contain affiliate links. If you buy through these links, you won't pay a penny more (in some cases it's cheaper), but I'll get a small commission.

If you would not like to use the links I've provided you may do a google search for the recommended item and go through their website directly.

This book is dedicated to your future body.

CONTENTS

ACKNOWLEDGEMENTS

Mum and Dad – You encouraged me to start my journey of becoming a personal trainer and have always been there to support me my whole life. I couldn't have asked for any better parents.

Colette Mason – This book simply would not be possible without the help from my friend Colette. She took what was a jumble of mish-mashed writing on a Microsoft Word document and helped me create the masterpiece that it is today.

Dan John – You may never read this book, but your wisdom and knowledge has helped me develop into the trainer I am today.

Tony Boutagy – You are another big influence on the trainer I have become. You are constantly challenging me to grow physically and mentally and to always improve my knowledge.

Abi Lemon – Thank you for helping me create the cover and design for this book! I know you didn't have much to work with when I first came to you (and it may have felt like pulling teeth from what was inside my head) but you made it work!

Greg Fidgeon – Thank you for taking the time to edit my book and make it "readable" as opposed to having 38,000 jumbled up words.

All of my friends, clients and followers – I wouldn't be where I am without the people who follow me on social media, without my clients who chose me over the thousands of other trainers in the world, and to my friends who've always encouraged me.

Honestly, I am so grateful for the support I have in my life and I feel like I'm one of the luckiest people around.

FOREWORD

In years past, the personal trainer was your stereotypical 6ft 6in, tight t-shirt-wearing bodybuilder (or the Lycra-clad female equivalent), where the advice given for training and nutrition would be based upon what worked for him (or her) and was often passed down from bodybuilder to apprentice, bodybuilder to apprentice.

Success and expertise in the modern era of personal training relies less on the Hulk-esque physique and nothing from the folk lore of our predecessors. It is now firmly based in scientific knowledge from across several fields which encompass physiology, biomechanics, nutrition, lifestyle medicine and exercise programming.

It is one thing to have a command of all these topics, but to be able to communicate these complexities in a way that can be understood and applied by non-professionals is a real art and skill – and one that Tyson Brown has mastered.

In this wonderful book, Tyson will lead you on a journey through the world of fasting, exercise and lifestyle management, providing the reader with usable advice on what to eat, how to fast and lifestyle tips to improve sleep and manage the inevitable ups and downs we have on our quest to improved health, vitality and fitness.

Applying Tyson's wisdom will transform your life. Today is a great day to begin the adventure.

Tony Boutagy, Ph.D,
Sports scientist and exercise physiologist

www.tonyboutagy.com

INTRODUCTION

ABOUT ME

Hello!

I'm Tyson Brown and I'm a fitness geek. I'm not shredded to the bone and I'm not a 100kg (200lbs) muscle man. I'm a normal guy who loves fitness, fun and getting shit done.

When I was growing up, I was the average kid. I never got picked first for the rugby team and I never got to represent the school for anything exciting.

I basically spent my time playing Xbox Live with my friends and eating lot of food. When I was about 16 years old, I started to become more aware of my body and I wasn't happy with how I looked. I'd be embarrassed to take my shirt off and I couldn't even do a proper push up. That's when I decided to join the gym and start taking care of my health and fitness.

Slowly over time my body started to change and I started losing fat. I started feeling good about myself and people started to compliment me. Once I was able to change my own body, I then wanted to help other people do the same. I was miserable in my job at the time (truck mechanic) and all I used to do was talk health and fitness. People around me were telling me I should become a trainer and so I thought I'd do it on the side. I got my Certificate IV in Personal Training, moved to the big city of Sydney (where I only knew one person) and decided to dive in head first.

Four years later on this journey and I still love every moment of it. Being able to teach people how they can transform their body and improve their health is one of the most satisfying things in the world.

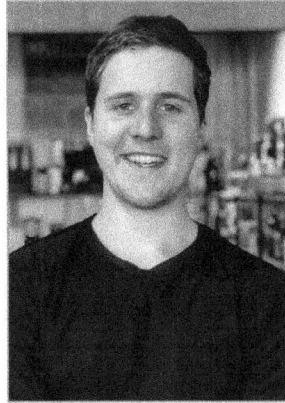

I love helping people transform their bodies because after four years of doing it − I've become pretty good at it.

(This is the part where I brag).

One of my goals is to become one of the best trainers in Australia − if not the world. I'm always looking to learn more and more about my craft so that I'm able to help people (like you) achieve their goals faster and, more importantly, stick to them in the long term.

I do this by learning from the best people in the industry. I travel around the world to be mentored and take courses on everything from fitness and nutrition to psychology. Right now, I am a personal trainer in Sydney, Australia, and I also coach clients online.

In 2016, I was the only Australian to be mentored Alwyn Cosgrove, who is one of the top ten gym owners in America. Over the years, I've obtained many qualifications and certifications from courses in exercise and nutrition. These include Precision Nutrition Coach, Food As Medicine at Monash University, Eat To Perform, Boutagy Fitness Institute, Underground Strength Coach, and Functional Movement Screening to name just a few.

I've trained TV actors including Max Ehlrich and fashion bloggers such as Samuel Wines. I've have also been published and written for various websites such as the PTDC, GymJunkies, Smallbiz magazine, Be Healthy Now and many more.

As well as writing, I also love being on camera. You've probably seen me pop up here or there in your Facebook or Instagram feed.

WHY I WROTE THIS BOOK

I know what it's like to wake up and feel deflated when you look in the mirror and don't like what you see, especially when you think you're doing everything right.

I was fed up with not being able to find a clear and practical book for helping people to lose weight both in the short and long term. There are plenty of diet books, but none of them are sustainable. They all seem to tell you that a certain food like dairy or carbs are evil, or that you can never have sugar again.

The exercise books are either tailored to bodybuilders or athletes – and you're neither of those. You're not looking to become the next Arnold Schwarzenegger.

The common advice is to spread out six meals a day and to train in the gym daily – and that's just unrealistic for most people.

I wanted to be able to share the methods that I've used on myself and my clients to help more people all over the world and I felt like it was time to get the knowledge out of my head on to paper.

I want to help as many people as possible to be able to lose fat now and, more importantly, keep it off forever!

I want to show you that you can still have the good quality of life you want without having to sacrifice going out with your friends.

I'm also going to show you the best exercises that don't take a lot of time and are the foundation for building nice lean muscle.

This book is here to break myths and share with you the truth you really need to hear about how to lose weight, keep it off, build lean muscle and improve your overall health and fitness.

Being healthy and fit doesn't mean you're surviving, it means you're thriving and I'm going to show you how to thrive in life.

WHO THIS BOOK IS FOR

This book is for the overworked guy who has tried the typical weight-loss diets, who's trained in the gym and who's been doing everything they think is right, but still isn't seeing results.

If you're sick of eating six small meals a day of nothing but chicken, broccoli and brown rice, and still not seeing that stubborn lower belly fat disappear then this is the book for you.

Follow the advice in this book and discover how to get rid of that belly flab once and for all.

WHAT THIS BOOK COVERS

This book is broken up into three parts and they are all as important as each other.

The first section is all about intermittent fasting and nutrition because this is the basis of your success. If you don't put the right types of food in your body – or put in too much or too little – you are not going to get the results you desire.

You'll learn about the right foods you should be eating, how to follow an intermittent fasting lifestyle and how you can create meal plans.

You'll also be shown the best strategies for meal preparation, food shopping and storage.

The second part of the book is about exercise. Lifting weights, doing cardio, improving your mobility and just leading an active lifestyle goes hand-in-hand with eating well and changing your body for the better. Exercise will improve your posture, your energy, the way you look and feel, and reduce the risk of many diseases.

You will also learn how you can train in a gym or at home, depending on your situation.

Building a lean physique doesn't just require using weights. You will learn different styles of training such as high intensity interval training (HIIT), low intensity steady state (LISS) and non-exercise activity thermogenesis (NEAT) activities (you'll learn more about these and what the terms mean later on) and a whole lot more. Cardio is extremely important for overall health and longevity.

The third section is lifestyle.

We always think about exercise and eating, but even though it sets the tone for how we live, people often forget to look at their lifestyle. Work, friends, family, where you live, how you sleep, and your stress levels – all these things come into play and influence how you do things and your success at being healthier.

The people you hang out with can convince you to have another drink, or five! Your lack of sleep can cause you to gain more fat around your midsection and become more insulin resistant.

Your co-workers bringing in a different type of cake every day because it's someone's birthday can determine whether you lose weight or not.

All of these factors need to be accounted for because they make up a major part of your day. Learning how to take control of your lifestyle will enable you to achieve some amazing results.

I'm going to teach you not only how to survive, but to thrive.

What if you could live an extra one, three, five or ten years? What if you could avoid having aches, pains and joint replacements? What if you could be 80 and still exercise, walk without a cane and still be able to wipe your own ass?

If you take care of your fitness now you have the potential to do all of that. The truth is some things may have to change.

Let me give you an example from a client of mine, Josef.

JOSEF – A SUCCESS STORY

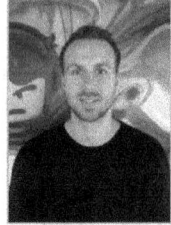

I wanted to lose weight and become healthier and so I bought a gym membership. I had all of the intentions to go, but work always got the best of me. A year later, I realised I hadn't stepped in the gym once since I purchased the membership.

I was ready to quit the gym, but they wanted to keep me around, so they offered me a personal training session to encourage me.

At first, I was hesitant but I thought, 'What the hell, why not?' After having a few sessions in the gym and realising how tough they were, I realised I needed to commit to it. I had to change what I ate and when I ate, but I never completely took away the foods I loved.

I started to become more aware about the foods I was eating and how they made me feel. I also started making the gym a morning habit to stick to it. I cut down my drinking but didn't stop it completely because I like to socialise with mates and I am also taking out clients for work. I got into a good workout routine; a combination of LISS, HIIT and weight training.

After about eight months of following the strategies laid out in this book, I had completely transformed my body.

I lost a lot of belly fat and I had been able to see my abs for the first time in a very long time.

Of course, I had some hiccups along the way and I could have achieved my goals faster if I wanted to, but I realised that this is a marathon and not a sprint.

I wanted to get lean and stay lean for the rest of my life, not just for three months of summer. I achieved that by following the exact strategies you're going to learn."

This book is called Ditch The Diet because it's based on living an intermittent fasting lifestyle while also having a busy life.

That is the foundation of this book. It doesn't mean you're going to achieve your goals super-fast because what's quick to one person might be something very different to the next.

My goal is to show you how to go from point A to point Z in the quickest way possible based on what quick is to you – whether that is two months or two years.

All of the instructions are laid out for you. You just have to follow them.

RESOURCES

I have created a great big folder of goodies for you to go with some of the material I mention in the book. These can be downloaded by going to the resources section at the back of the book (page 169).

KEEP IN TOUCH

Please make sure you share your success stories with me and your progress photos, so you can help other people with their motivation by showing them that they too can also make amazing changes. If you're struggling or facing challenges let me know. I've not written this book for me, I've written it for you.

If you want even more help, we can work together online. Just go to www.tysonbrown.com.au/online-coaching for more details.

THIS ISN'T JUST FOR FAT LOSS

If you don't want to lose weight but just want to learn how to optimise your body, you can still practice intermittent fasting.

Right now, I'm not trying to lose weight. I'm actually trying to gain muscle. I still follow intermittent fasting because it allows me to get the most out of my body, physically and mentally.

Intermittent fasting isn't some fad diet that's going away anytime soon. You're going to be seeing some amazing research on the long-term and short-term health benefits of intermittent fasting, so you too can see why it's so powerful.

My job isn't to just help you lose weight and get lean, it is to help you live longer and have a better quality of life.

Receiving messages from people and having clients tell me how much I've helped change their lives gives me a massive high. But I get an even a bigger high when I think about the long-term impact I'm having on their health and fitness.

If I can add another one or three years to your life, if I can be the person who dramatically reduces the chance of you having diabetes, if I can be the guy who has allowed you to still be able to get off the toilet by yourself at 80 instead of having someone do it for you, then that's when I know I've really done my job.

How will I be able to know if I've helped you do that? To be honest, I have no idea. But somewhere deep down, I just know that I'm making an impact and that's why I love what I do.

PS. If this book does help you in any way, please send me a message to let me know. You guys are my oxygen and I love hearing feedback as to how I've helped.

Even if it's just one small thing that you take away from this book or you liked a certain part, just send me a quick message to:

tyson@tysonbrown.com.au

I read every email and I will reply to you.

1
KNOWING YOUR 'WHY'

Why did you pick up this book? What led you to grab this off the shelf? I know the title grabbed your attention, but what else intrigued you?

Is it because you think this "non-diet book" might be the answer to your problems? Do you think this might be the book that will help you get rid of that stubborn belly fat once and for all?

Before getting into this book and learn my methods, really think about what you want to get from reading this.

Is it a short-term fix to just get rid of your belly fat as quickly as possible? Or is it to be able to transform your life, be healthier, live longer and be there for your kids when you're older?

Do you want to lose weight because your doctor said you're creeping towards becoming diabetic?

Do you want to feel good with your shirt off when you're on the beach?

Or do you want to make sure you're at your daughter's wedding in 20 or 30 years' time?

There's no right or wrong answer because everyone is different, but you need to know what you want and, more importantly, why you want to achieve that goal.

Think about this in three time frames. What do you want to achieve in the next 12 weeks? What do you want to achieve in the next three years? And what do you want to achieve in the very long term?

Most likely, your goal for 12 weeks is going to be based on appearance and there's nothing wrong with that. But you also need to think about this from a long-term perspective.

This isn't a short-term diet, it's a lifestyle change to implement and you've got to think about why you would want to stick to a healthier lifestyle in the long term.

It's easy to say you want to be healthier, but if your actions don't line up with your short-term and long-term visions then you won't achieve your goals.

Being in alignment with your goals is what will stop you from skipping the gym or from binging on a Friday night because you've had a crappy day at work.

Once you've thought about what you want, now ask yourself why?

TASK: DIG DEEP TO FIND YOUR 'WHY'

A good practice to do is to ask yourself "why?" five times in order to really find the deep answer.

For example: I want to lose weight.

Why 1: Because I hate having this stomach.

Why 2: Because when all my friends go swimming at the beach, I am hesitant or embarrassed to take my shirt off.

Why 3: Because it's very embarrassing to have all of this extra belly fat and I feel ashamed.

Why 4: Because then I feel like everyone is judging me and it looks like I can't take care of my body.

Why 5: Because I don't take care of my body and I know that if I don't make a change soon I'm going to feel embarrassed for the rest of my life. I don't want that. I want to be able to feel confident with my shirt off.

BOOM!

Now you've just figured out why you really want something and it connects to an emotion.

This book will provide you with practical "how to" information for not only losing stubborn belly fat but also transforming the way you live so you can build that lean body you've been craving.

Even more importantly, so you can live longer too.

Knowing your 'Why' is going to keep you on track when the times get tough – and at the start, it will be tough.

Change is hard, but change is also good. Change is what makes us grow and, I promise you, this type of change will be the best you've ever experienced.

Once you've worked out your 'Why', you need to write this and your goal down on a piece of paper or type it up and print it out.

Have it on display somewhere you can see it every day. This is going to remind you of what you're working towards and why.

It's easy to fall off the bandwagon when things get hard, but if you have that piece of paper to remind you of what you're working towards and why you're doing it, it's going to motivate you and keep you on track when things get tough.

I know what you're thinking and I thought the same thing at first. "Why do I need to do this woo-woo stuff? I just want to lose weight, now." And I get it; of course you want to lose weight now. We all do. But this isn't just a short-term fix, this is a lifestyle change and if you want to stick to a healthier lifestyle then you'd better have a reason why.

Stand for something or fall for anything.

SHORT-TERM GOALS

You now know your 'Why' and what your goals are, so it's time to put the stepping stones to getting there in place.

The next thing you need to do is set yourself a 12-week goal.

Why 12? Because you won't see much change after a month, but your friends and family will notice in eight weeks and once the 12 weeks are up, you'll look in the mirror and think, 'Shit, who's that person looking back at me?'

Another reason a 12-week goal is so important is because most of us are short-term thinkers. Sure, losing 30kg (66lbs) this year would be great. But you want to start shedding fat now, right?

Twelve weeks is a short enough time frame to be able to go hard and think of the actions you need to take to achieve your goal.

We're going to use SMART goal-setting for your 12-week target to hone in on exactly what you want and how to get there. Here's how it works.

THE SMART SYSTEM

S (Specific): The goal you're going to set needs to be specific. Losing weight is general and is not going to motivate you, but losing 8kg (18lbs) in 12 weeks is a more specific goal.

Once you have specified your target, you then need to write down why you want to lose that amount of weight in that time. Is it because there's an event coming up? Or is it because this is part of your long-term goal to lose 30kg (66lbs) this year?

Making your goal more specific and clear will allow you to know exactly when you have achieved it.

M (Measurable): You need to be able to measure the progress you're making weekly and monthly. If you want to lose fat, you would measure it by weighing yourself on a scale, checking the notches on your belt, or doing body measurements and photos.

A (Attainable): Is your goal really attainable? One way to decide is to ask yourself if someone else has achieved what you want to before.

Have people lost weight before? Absolutely. Have people lost 8kg (18lbs) of body fat in 12 weeks? Yep.

Before writing down your goal, just look around to see if your goal is attainable in the time frame.

R (Realistic): A lot of people (including me), tend to overshoot what we can do in a short amount of time.

"I'm going to lose 20kg (45lbs) in 12 weeks!"

That is unrealistic and would be setting yourself up for failure. You need to think about what's going on in your life at that moment, how much time you're going to be able to dedicate to your goal and what's going to get in your way. Make it realistic.

As a guide, losing 0.25kg to 0.5kg (0.5lbs to 1lb) in a week is very realistic for most people.

T (Time bound): You've already got the timeline set up, which is 12 weeks. But you need to break that down into weekly and daily actionable steps and achievable goals.

Example of a non-smart goal:

This year I'm going to go to the gym and lose weight

Example of a smart goal:

Summer is getting closer and in the next three months I'm going to lose 5kg of body fat and weigh 70kg.

TASK: PREPARE TO SUCCEED

Now that you've set yourself a SMART goal, it's time to do some brainstorming. Get yourself another blank piece of paper and take some time to write down everything that you can think of that you need to do in order to prepare for and achieve your weekly and daily goals. This would include things like:

- buy gym membership
- weight train three times a week
- do meal prep once a week
- do an extra 30 minutes of walking every day
- go grocery shopping every Wednesday and Sunday
- buy frozen vegetables to keep at work

Can you see how this goal is becoming a clearer picture in your head? You've got the dials spinning and you know exactly what you need to do to get there.

This is a powerful tool once you get it right because you now have a road map of exactly where you need to go, how long you've got, how you're going to get there and the exact things you need to do every day.

The final thing you need to do is to write down the daily action steps in your calendar or journal, so you always know what you're doing tomorrow, the day after and in the week ahead.

Block out the times you're going to exercise and when you're going to do meal prep every week. When you put it in the calendar, you're not going to forget and miss a step.

ACTION STEPS

1. Take some time to think about your goals and why you want to achieve them.
2. Practice the 'Why?' method to find your deep, underlying reason.
3. Create a 12-week SMART goal.
4. Print out your goal and your 'Why' and display it where you can see it every day.
5. Write down everything you need to do in order to reach your goal.
6. Book out those daily to-dos in your calendar.

2
TRACKING PROGRESS

Tracking your progress is crucial because failing to do so will mean you don't know how you're doing and whether or not you're on the right track towards achieving your goal.

Three great ways to track your progress are through photos, using a body tape and using scales. Let's look at each of those in a bit more detail.

PHOTOS

Humans are visual creatures. We would much rather be able to see something to understand it and when it comes to making progress in the gym, one of the best ways is to take photos.

If you're looking at yourself in the mirror every day, the chances are you're not going to notice as much of a difference as you will with photos. You just get to see a very gradual change in the mirror, because the changes will be small and subtle every week.

But when you take monthly photos, you're able to look back and see if you've truly progressed (or if you haven't) and you will be able to see the most notable areas in which you've improved.

Whether you have improved or not, the photos are going to give you motivation to keep pushing.

Nothing feels better than being able to see progress and it will spur you on to achieve more.

On the flip side, nothing feels worse than realising that you're behind on your goals, which means it's time to adjust what you're doing to get back on track.

Lighting, camera angle and many other variables can change the way you look and give you a false reality (think about all of the people on the front of fitness magazines or on Instagram).

Photos don't lie if taken correctly. Make sure you're just in your under-wear and you're standing against a white wall in the same spot each time the pictures are taken. That way, there isn't any room for error.

Take four photos minimum – one from the front, one of you facing to the left, one of you facing to the right, and one of you facing the wall. Get someone else to take them if you need help.

One thing you might notice after a few months of weight training and healthy eating is that your posture is improving and you're standing taller. You might start to notice that you have more definition around your chest and less fat around your face.

Note: Don't expect miracles in a month. Your first two batches of photos probably won't show that much of a dramatic change and that's com-pletely normal.

It didn't take you one month to put all of your weight on, so don't expect it to all come back off in a month either.

Put a reminder in your calendar to take monthly photos and keep them somewhere you can compare them easily.

TAPE MEASURE

Measuring your body allows you to discover exactly where you're losing fat and whether you're losing it in the right areas.

You can measure as many points as you like, but here are the best areas to keep an eye on:

- waist
- hips
- legs (thighs)

- arms
- chest
- shoulders

That's pretty much all we tend to worry about and you don't want to be spending too much time measuring each and everybody part.

These areas are where you will store the most muscle and fat, so it's a good guide.

All of your measurements will go down when you're losing weight. People get discouraged when they see their chest, arms and shoulders go down half a centimetre, but you can't decide where you're losing fat from and you store fat all over your body.

The most important thing is you're seeing the waist and hip measurements decrease each time you measure. This is your goal in losing fat. Take you measurements once a month at the same time as your photos.

Body fat callipers can also be a useful tool if you know how to use them properly. They can be more accurate with measuring your body fat. If there is someone at your local gym who can do the measurements for you, then I'd suggest getting them to help. Otherwise the measuring tape will work just as well.

SCALES

You've probably heard that scales are evil and that you shouldn't be weighing yourself every day. If you have a very unhealthy relationship with your weight, then you probably shouldn't weigh yourself daily.

But if you don't have a problem, then doing a daily check-in is the best way to keep track of your running average weight and to give you real-time feedback week-by-week and day-by-day to know if you're heading in the right direction.

Waking up every morning, going to the bathroom and weighing yourself at the same time is going to give you a fairly accurate measure of what your weight actually is. It will fluctuate 0.5kg to 1kg (1lb to 2lbs) or more depending on factors such as a big dinner, how much water you drink, and how much salt you've had, etc.

Don't be too worried if you wake up one day and you're 1kg (2lbs) heavier all of a sudden. It doesn't mean you've just gained a kilo of fat. Usually, there's a reason behind it.

Instead of focusing on the day-to-day scale, it's good to look at it weekly to find out what your average weight is.

If you weigh yourself every day Monday to Sunday and your weight looks like this:

DAY	WEIGHT
Monday	70.0kg
Tuesday	71.6kg
Wednesday	70.0kg
Thursday	71.0kg
Friday	70.2kg
Saturday	72.0kg
Sunday	70.0kg

Combine all of those numbers together and divide it by seven. Your average weight is 70.6kg.

Knowing this will allow you to see week-by-week if the weight is going up or down and determine if you need adjustments.

When it comes to buying scales, just get a simple set of digital bathroom scales and make sure they're on a flat surface.

Don't buy those scales that claim they can tell you your body fat percentage. These can be inaccurate due to the amount of water you're holding and other factors. They're a waste of money and a normal set of bathroom scales will do the job you want.

TRACKING FOOD

You don't want to be counting calories in every meal for the rest of your life or measuring your macronutrients, but knowing how much food you're eating on a daily basis and coming to grips with how much you really eat is essential.

When you become more aware of what and when you're eating, you are going to be able to see patterns emerge and you can then make the changes necessary.

BRAD AND THE PHANTOM DOUGHNUTS

I had a client called Brad. Every day at work, his colleague would go out at about 3pm and buy a box of doughnuts for everyone in the office. Here's what he discovered...

"Without really thinking about it, I would just grab one or two and nibble away at them for the rest of the day. I was wondering why I couldn't lose weight and why I felt sluggish in the afternoon.

"It was only when I started tracking my food that I realised I was eating two sometimes three doughnuts daily and the impact they had.

"Two key things came about from the tracking. First, I discovered I was unconsciously eating food out of boredom. I thought it was occasional snacking, but it was every single day.

> *"Secondly, I got to understand just how many calories there are in not just the doughnuts, but in all the food I was eating (it turns out one doughnut is between 250 and 350 calories).*
>
> *"After becoming more aware of what was going on, I was able to make the changes to cut out the bad habits of late afternoon snacking by replacing the doughnuts with something less calorie dense and reduce the food I was eating overall."*

I suggest tracking your food using an app called MyFitnessPal. You can download this on your phone for free. Tracking your food to become more aware of everything that you are eating and drinking is a key step in losing that stubborn fat.

> ☑ **TIP:** Download my 'how to' guides on taking body measurements and photos. It's in the resources section.

ACTION STEPS

1. Set a reminder in your calendar every four weeks to take photos and body measurements.
2. Buy yourself a set of standard bathroom scales to weigh yourself every day and a body tape to track your measurements monthly.
3. Download the MyFitnessPal app to track your food.

PART ONE

INTERMITTENT FASTING

"I fast for greater physical and
mental efficiency"
- Plato -

3
WHAT IS INTERMITTENT FASTING?

You've probably heard the word "fasting" before. There are juice fasts, water fasts, daily fasts, and a lot of cultures follow different types of fasting.

But you may be less familiar with the idea of intermittent fasting. This is a broad term for various types of diets that cycle between a period of fasting and a period of non-fasting (or put simply, eating and not eating).

THREE TYPES OF FASTING

You're going to learn about three types of fasting that you can follow. They are one meal a day (OMAD), whole day fasting, and time-restricted eating (TRE).

Let's have a look at each of those in a bit more depth.

ONE MEAL A DAY (OMAD)

OMAD involves a 22 to 23-hour fasting period followed by one to two hours non-fasting.

The most popularised version of this is known as the Warrior Diet and was created by Ori Hofmekler.

The premise is that you would consume very few (if any) calories during the day and just eat one big meal. You would eat this at, say, around 6pm and it will be just a typical dinner.

For example: You might have three portions of lean protein, three to four fistfuls of vegetables, a large sweet potato for your carbohydrate source and a whole avocado for your healthy fats. You would drizzle over some olive oil over the top and add a shake with your meal to ensure you're eating enough. This could be a combination of a small handful nuts, half a cup of oats, one cup of milk and a medium banana.

Eating just one meal a day can be very difficult, especially if you've never done fasting before. But if you have a big appetite (like me) then this can be a useful strategy to avoid over-eating and to help restrict your calories.

I do OMAD on the first Sunday of every month to give my digestion a bit of a rest, reset my hunger cues and just remind myself that I'm not going to die if I don't eat for 24 hours.

This method is more for someone who has super-hectic days at work and just can't fit any time to eat food into their day, someone who has a problem with eating too much food or you can do it once a month to give your digestion a rest.

WHOLE-DAY FASTING

With this method, you specify various ratios of fasting to non-fasting days. You may have heard of the 5:2 Diet, which was created by Krista Varady's group that did the initial research and then popularised by Dr. Michael Mosley. People eat freely for five days and on the other two, consume 400 to 500 calories for women or 500 to 600 for men.

I'm going to share with you a slightly different approach in this book that is tailored more towards a person who wants to combine fasting and lifting weights.

This approach to intermittent fasting is called the Deficit Day System and was thought up by one of my mentors, Tony Boutagy. It is more focused on exercise and building muscle.

With the Deficit Day System, you create major calorie deficits on several days during the week and then on the other days you "eat normally". On deficit days, you're restricting your calories to about a third of what you would you usually eat.

The average male burns about 2,400 calories a day. This means that for the deficit days you would only be eating 800 calories and the majority of those calories would come from protein.

The reason you want most of these calories coming from protein is that you want to protect or even build lean muscle and you need protein in order to do that.

Your deficit days would fall on the days you train with weights because weight training is also protective of muscle. When you lift weights, you're sending signals throughout your body to use protein and carbs more efficiently, so it goes to your muscles.

Typically, you would only eat two meals on these days. You will skip breakfast, have an early lunch between 11am and 12pm and then a dinner at 5pm to 6pm.

Keep your first meal small and light, and then have more calories around dinner time.

Lunch could be something as simple as two scoops of protein powder with water.

Then your dinner would be a big lean serving of protein (fillet of white fish, chicken breast, a piece of steak, etc.) a lot of leafy green vegetables and salads, and a small serving of starchy carbs (think sweet potato or some type of legumes).

That's basically all you would have for the day because you're restricted to only 800 calories – and when you find out how many calories those foods contain you will be very surprised.

To follow this program, pick two days during the week when you're going to do weight training and make them deficit days.

In this example, we'll pick Monday and Thursday. Having a day at the start of the week and one in the middle will mean you're more likely to stick to it.

You're less likely to go out for breakfast since it's not a weekend and you're not going to go out for dinner with mates since it's not a Friday night. You're also less likely to have lunch commitments on a Monday.

Let's take a closer look at those deficit days.

You wake up and train at 7am, and then you're on your way to work by 8.30am.

Have something like a black coffee, black tea, green tea or sparkling water (anything with no calories) to keep hunger at bay.

At 11.45am you have your first meal, which is a shake consisting of two scoops of chocolate protein powder. Then have another tea at around 3pm to keep the hunger cravings away.

You have dinner at 5.30pm, which is chilli con carne, and you finish eating by 6pm.

> ☑ **TIP:** I've created a bunch of tasty recipes for you to download. It's in the resources section.

For the next two days, you go back to eating at a normal time that suits you and following the 90/10 approach of eating. This means 90 per cent of your intake of the day should be whole, nutritious, unprocessed foods and ten per cent on a few pieces of chocolate, etc.

This method works well for people who have busy days and don't really worry about food. If you struggle with trying to manage calorie intake day-to-day then this would be a better option because you're putting yourself in a big deficit for only two to three days during the week and don't really have to focus too much during the rest of the week.

You will get some cravings for the foods you want at first, but you're just going to have to resist.

Remember, it's only a few days during the week and one thing that is very helpful to overcome your cravings is telling yourself you can have a normal day tomorrow. Then, when it is your "normal day", the craving will be gone anyways.

I really suggest you follow Tony's work and learn as much as you can from him at www.tonyboutagy.com.

TIME-RESTRICTED EATING (TRE)

The final method you need to be aware of is TRE, which involves a set daily fasting period and shortened eating window of three to ten hours.

This is my favourite way of intermittent fasting and I follow the most common approach – 16:8. This means that you fast for 16 hours each day and eat all of your daily calories during the remaining eight hours.

This diet has been widely popularised thanks to Martin Berkhan and the diet is known as Leangains. It's the most popular method for those who lift weights as food is very important for muscle growth.

Food is anabolic and you need to give your body enough nutrients and fuel to signal muscle growth.

If you're going for long periods of not eating, then you're not signalling to your body that you want to build lean muscle.

With this system, you have a window every day when you're eating and one when you're not – but you're still getting food into your body daily.

Here are the different types of TRF that people use:

FASTING WINDOW	EATING WINDOW
14	10
16	8
18	6
20	4
22	2 (OMAD)

You can go for longer periods without eating, but then you're falling into one of the other types of fasting.

If you think this would be a great starting point for you because you would rather eat food every day, start with the 14-hour fasting period and ten-hour eating window just to get used to it.

The longer you go without food at first, the harder it's going to be and you don't want to set yourself up for failure.

TOO MUCH TOO SOON – A FUNNY STORY

I had been doing 16:8 for about a year and I decided to challenge myself on my first 23-hour fast by doing OMAD and eat all of my calories in one meal.

I was a young personal trainer who was really active and burned a lot of calories, meaning I needed to eat about 3,500 a day.

I don't eat a lot of junk food and decided to try and eat what I usually would.

What I discovered was that trying to eat 3,500 calories in one meal from whole foods is extremely hard. After about 40 minutes of chewing and eating, it wasn't fun anymore and I started to get stomach cramps. My body was telling me to stop eating, but I just kept going because I thought I had to get all of my calories in or I'd lose muscle.

I didn't get to eat all of my food because I just simply couldn't fit more in. I had to sit down and just breathe extremely heavily for about ten minutes before I could get up.

My stomach felt like it was about to explode and I thought I was going to have to go to the hospital from eating too much.

I slowly got up, made my way over to the couch and proceeded to lay down in agony because that's all I could do.

I kept thinking, 'Why did I do this? This was a terrible mistake'. I was incapacitated on the couch for the rest of the night.

I ended up falling asleep but kept waking up during the night in agony. The next morning and realised two things:

1. *If you're going to do OMAD, you might want to eat more food either the day before or the day after, so you aren't trying to force feed yourself in one meal.*
2. *Work up to something slowly. Don't just go from a 16-hour fast to a 23-hour one straight away. Work up to it.*

WHAT CAN YOU HAVE WHILE FASTING?

There is a lot of debate about what can be consumed during the fast because certain foods still contain "zero calories", such as sugar-free drinks, teas, black coffee, chewing gum, etc.

The problem with sugar-free drinks and gums is that they're still telling the body that there's going to be food coming, because of the sweet taste. This can cause certain functions in your body to start happening (like increasing your hunger or releasing insulin), which we don't want.

There has been a lot more research recently on how our bodies have an internal clock run by our organs, and once our organs start having to work then our body is no longer in a "fasted state".

This means that when coffees, teas or anything that has to be metabolised is consumed, you're no longer in a fasted state.

But since your goal is to use intermittent fasting to lose fat and to make it work with *your* lifestyle, the information above will not apply. You can have your sugar free gums, drinks, black coffees and teas.

Here's what I recommend. From the last bite of your food at dinner time, consume nothing but water for a minimum of 12 hours.

After those 12 hours, you have the options of consuming:

- black coffee
- black/green/herbal tea
- water with a squirt of lemon or lime
- pre-workout that has fewer than ten calories
- Essential Amino Acids (EAAS)

After that – depending on which of the styles of fasting you follow – you would eat on your schedule.

Why a minimum of 12 hours? Because this allows the health benefits of fasting to start kicking in.

Let me give you an example of a typical day for me:

TIME	WEIGHT
07;00	Black coffee while training clients
07;45	Training session
09;00	Meal one
12;30	Meal two
16;30	Meal three
17;00	Fasting begins

The reason I have my dinner so early is that I like to have my coffee in the morning and I want to fast for a minimum of 14 hours.

Another reason I like to have dinner early is that I train clients in the evenings and I don't want to wait until I get home at 8pm to scoff down a big meal right before bed.

Eating dinner further away from going to sleep has also been shown to help improve your sleep quality, because your body isn't focused on trying to digest food.

After reviewing these three styles of fasting, the basic premise is that there are extended periods of time when you're not going to be eating and instead consuming nothing but water, black coffee and black tea.

In a way, this book is a "choose your own adventure" because everyone is different when it comes to the types of eating styles.

You have to decide which fasting style will suit you best based on your eating habits, your work and your lifestyle.

Maybe it's easier for you to eat one day and not eat another day, or maybe it's more suitable to eat on a daily basis.

There is no "optimal" way to practice intermittent fasting, the most important thing is that you just take action and do it.

Pick one option that you think will suit your lifestyle the best and set a goal for one month to try it.

WHY WOULD ANYONE DO THIS?

That's a good question. When I first heard about this type of diet I thought it was complete BS!

I thought if I didn't eat every few hours I would lose my muscle mass, all of my gym "gains" would disappear and my workouts would be a waste of time.

Boy was I wrong.

Let's think about this logically. Back in our ancestral days, we didn't have access to a fridge or a bowl of oats as soon as we woke up.

We had to hunt and kill our food or go foraging for it.

We could go days and weeks before we got food again. This meant that when we did get food, we would eat a lot because we never knew when our next meal would come.

Evolution got clever and when we didn't eat for long periods of time we learned to tap into our bodies' stored fuel sources (fats and carbs), which would give us energy in times when we couldn't eat.

Do you think our bodies would start burning muscle as soon as we didn't have food for three hours? If that were the case, you and I wouldn't be alive right now.

Humans are designed to go for long periods without food and still stay alive.

Don't try intermittent fasting for a few days or a week and decide it's not for you because you didn't get "ripped". Results don't happen that quickly. It's not like you see on Instagram.

Another reason I suggest trying it for a minimum of a month is that it will take time to adopt a new style of eating, and there will be times where you're hungry.

You're changing the way you eat, but your body is used to how often you're eating at the moment.

If you're eating dinner at 8pm every night and you wake up and have breakfast at 6am, your body knows this and has certain cues and hormones that are released around these times.

Do you ever notice how you get hungry when it's time to eat? That's your body clock saying, "Hey, it's 6am and its breakfast time. It's time to feed me."

These habits can be changed, but the body won't adapt to it straight away.

If you go from eating at 6am and not having your first meal until 10am then your body is going to be telling you to eat at 6am for the next few days until it gets used to the new eating habit.

So, you will start to get hungry.

Usually it will take a few weeks for your body to get used to the new routine, which is why it's so important not to give up so early.

I'm going to share strategies on how you can keep hunger at bay when you're first getting started.

RESULTS TAKE TIME

You can't get the body you want in a week or a month. Think about how long it took you to put on weight.

It wasn't like one day you woke up and were like, "Oh, I'm fat and my belt won't fit anymore." It slowly and surely crept on day-by-day, and you have to use the same approach when trying to get the weight off.

Slowly and surely, day-by-day, you will put in these new eating and lifestyle habits until they're ingrained in your brain – until they're so hardwired that it's a pain not to do follow this lifestyle.

Having been following this way of eating for more than four years, it's actually harder for me not to do it as opposed to doing it, and I want this to be the same way for you.

Aside from the physical changes that take time, there are a lot of other benefits that you will begin to notice in a few days such as:

- mental clarity
- more energy
- less brain fog
- more productivity
- better skin
- better sleep
- increased insulin sensitivity
- increased brain derived neurotrophic factor (BDNF)

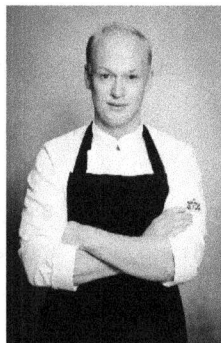

ACTION STEPS

1. Out of the three types of fasting I described above, pick the one that you think will suit your lifestyle best.
2. Try to drink nothing but water for the first 12 hours of your fast.
3. Only consume black coffee, green tea, black tea, herbal teas, water with a squeeze of lemon or lime, or anything else with zero calories during your fasting window.
4. Commit to sticking to this way of eating for a minimum of three to four weeks.

4
WHAT TO EAT

How many diets have you tried in the past and managed to stick to them? If you're like me, you've tried a truckload and they've all failed.

Why?

Firstly, they are too restrictive. Most diet books tell you to cut out this food and that, or only eat chicken and brown rice every lunch for the rest of your life.

When you first start a diet, you get really excited and follow exactly what is recommended. You steam all of your chicken and broccoli, you boil your brown rice and you throw away all of the "bad stuff".

Six weeks later you're staring that at that God-damned boiled chicken again at lunch while your co-worker is scoffing down a juicy burger and you can't take it anymore.

So, what usually happens is you fall off the wagon because it's simply unsustainable.

The second reason those diets tend to fail is your environment.

Does any of this sound familiar? Your friends or family want to go out to a pub/restaurant/cafe for a meal and you just go along and eat whatever just so you're not being unsociable.

Or your spouse/housemate/kids have food in the house that you're not supposed to eat, but you come home from a stressful day at work to see the block of chocolate in the fridge or a bag of potato chips in the pantry and you just go balls to the wall.

When these "hiccups" happen, you start to beat yourself up and think, 'Fuck it, it's too hard. I'm just going back to how I was.'

All that progress you've made through hard work and dieting for six or nine weeks and then you just throw it all away. (Don't worry I've been there too.)

This is why the intermittent fasting approach works so well; because it isn't a short-term diet, it is a lifestyle approach to eating and living. If you're looking to get ripped in six weeks, then I'm sorry to inform you but it's going to take longer than that.

One thing I pride myself on is not restricting myself from food. If I want to go out to dinner with my friends once a week and eat something "naughty", I will.

I used to really beat myself up about this, but after a few years and learning from some of my mentors, I came to understand that life is meant to be enjoyed and you should go out and experience things.

The principle I suggest you follow is the 90/10 approach.

Ninety per cent of the food you eat should be whole nutritious food that's not packed and processed, and you can then have some leeway in the remaining ten per cent of your diet.

If you are eating three meals a day following the 16:8 fasting approach, that's 21 meals a week. That means two meals a week should be "treat meals".

You'll notice I said "treat meals" and not "cheat meals" because you're not really cheating yourself.

Cheating means that you scoff down a whole pizza, a large Coke and a block of chocolate in 30 minutes acting like it's the last meal you're ever going to be able to eat and thinking you can get away with it.

What usually happens after you stuff your gullet?

You feel guilty, sick, you have breakouts, and you throw your weight-loss progress back two weeks and have to build it up all over again.

Then you make some progress and its cheat meal time again. You wind up with this weight stall plateau and wonder why?

A "treat meal" on the other hand is taking time to enjoy what you're eating and not feel guilty about it afterwards.

A treat is eating half a pizza instead of a whole one, a small Coke instead of a large, and eating it with your family on a Friday night and actually enjoying it instead of hiding in the fridge so no one sees you.

I haven't touched soft drink or pizza in years because I just don't enjoy how it makes me feel, but I'm not telling you to be like me.

I still go out with friends and family for my "treat meal" but I make sure it's good quality food and not something crappy.

THE MYTH OF EATING HEALTHY

Eating healthily isn't the magic pill to weight loss.

Just because you eat healthy food it does not mean that you will lose weight.

There are a lot of diets that tell you it doesn't matter what you eat and as long as you follow their approach you will lose weight – but that's complete bullshit.

Some people say that if you just listen to your body you will know exactly what you need. That's bullshit too. This is because the way we've been brought up affects our relationship with food.

THE LAW OF THERMODYNAMICS

If you consume more energy than you burn during the day, then you will not lose weight. It's plain and simple.

There have been studies that show that if you are put in a chamber and given less food than you need for the day, you're going to lose weight.

The truth is most people (myself included) are quite terrible at accurately measuring how much we eat over a day and a week.

We forget foods – usually the bad foods we eat like the birthday cake at work, the late-night snacks and those few extra wines after a stressful day. We tend to only remember the good stuff.

Intermittent fasting isn't going to change this.

Just because I'm writing a whole book on this lifestyle doesn't mean you're going to magically start losing weight if you reduce the amount of time you eat.

If you still consume a lot of calorie-dense food in that shorter time span, whether those extra calories come from fistfuls of healthy nuts and muesli or a McDonald's cheeseburger, then you will gain weight.

FOOD QUALITY STILL MATTERS

Just because you can lose weight by eating less energy than you burn, it doesn't mean get away with still eating fast food and takeaway every day. That's just stupid.

Food quality is incredibly important for a long and healthy life, for boosting your mood and energy, for certain hormone and enzyme functions, and for a better quality of life overall.

All of the micronutrients you get from whole, unprocessed foods will do wonders for your body and you will feel the difference.

Go and eat a large Big Mac, fries and a Coke one day and see how you feel afterwards.

The next day, go and eat the exact same amount of calories from baked potatoes, a good steak and steamed vegetables with avocado.

The way those foods act in your body are going to be completely different and the way you feel will speak for itself.

This is why I'm such a big advocate of the 90/10 approach – because there will be times where you will want to go out with friends and family or eat a bag of chips on occasion.

THERE WILL BE SLIP-UPS!

Here's a quick reality check. You're going to mess up. That's a fact.

One day you might not sleep as well as you usually do and you give into some cravings, or you have some friends who manage to talk you into a big night of binge drinking and greasy food.

We've all been there. The most important thing is to not beat yourself up when this happens.

Remember this is a lifestyle and not a diet – you didn't "ruin it". If you eat shitty food, you can do a 24-hour fast the next day, drink nothing but water and get straight back on track.

One day is a tiny blip on your lifetime journey.

The worst thing you can think is say: "Well it's Wednesday and I've just messed up my diet. What's the point? I might as well wait until next week/month/year."

That's where you make the situation worse because the deeper the hole you dig for yourself, the harder it's going to be to get back out.

Remember that an object in motion stays in motion. You can use that positively or negatively, it's your choice.

WHAT DO YOU EAT?

People say all the time: "Come on Tyson, just tell me what I should and shouldn't be eating. Give me a diet plan to follow."

Do you really want to be eating the exact same food day in and day out for the rest of your life?

Instead of giving you a specific meal plan, I want to give you a guide and let you be the creator of your own meals.

> ☑ **TIP:** I've created a bunch of tasty recipes for you to download. It's in the resources.

Here's the principle: At every meal you want to make sure you're consuming some good quality food from each macronutrient (protein, carbs and fats). How much of each? That's where the beauty of your hands comes in.

PROTEIN

Protein is the most important macronutrient to focus on first. If you want to gain lean muscle, prevent hunger, avoid losing muscle, stay fuller for longer and keep a whole bunch of important functions that happen in your body, you must make protein your friend.

If you're eating three meals a day while following intermittent fasting, you want to make sure you consume two palm-sized servings of lean protein at each meal.

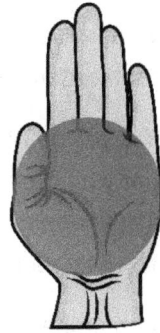

If you're eating two meals, then you would want to be consuming more. The goal of making sure you're eating enough protein is aiming for 2g per kilogram of body weight (0.8g per 1lb).

So, if you weigh 70kg (155lbs) you would aim to get 140g of protein every day – 70 x 2g = 140.

This doesn't mean you only need to eat 140g of chicken breast or steak because that's not all protein either.

A 100g chicken breast or steak is roughly 20-22g of protein, so you would need a lot more than 100g to reach your 140g goal.

That's why I like to go off palm-sized servings. Two palm-sized servings of lean meat is going to put you at around 40-50g of protein and if you're having three meals that means you're going to be consuming roughly 150g of protein, which will be ideal.

Protein should come from a variety of different sources and you should not just eat chicken breast all day every day. The gut likes variety and eating the same thing gets very boring very quickly.

VEGETABLES AND SALADS

Vegetables and salads also need to be an essential part of your diet.

They are chock-full of vitamins and minerals that your body needs to not only survive, but to thrive. If you want to be at your best, feel great and keep the fat off, then vegetables and salads are a must.

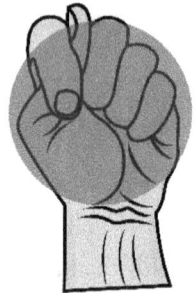

You're not 12 years old anymore; you need to learn to eat your damn vegetables. Don't complain that you just don't like them. There are so many varieties out there that you can – and must – find a few that you love.

Remember the first time you tried alcohol? You didn't say: "Hmmm, beer is the best-tasting thing in the world?" or "This vodka sure does go down a treat."

I don't think you did.

Don't expect all vegetables to taste amazing the first time you try them. And remember, there are different ways you can cook them too (yes, you can do more with broccoli than just steam it).

Use two fist-sized servings of vegetables at each meal to make sure you're getting enough.

FATS

There are different types of fats and you need to be aware of how much you're consuming, but having them in your diet is vital. Healthy fats aren't the devil and you shouldn't avoid them.

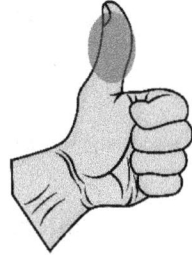

Fats are essential for certain functions in the body (including producing hormones such as testosterone) so you want to make sure you're getting the right types.

THE FOUR TYPES OF FATS

- saturated fats
- polyunsaturated fats
- monounsaturated fats
- trans fats (bad fats)

Polyunsaturated and monounsaturated fats

Your main sources of fats should be coming from a combination of poly and monounsaturated fats. These types of fats come from grass-fed meat, eggs, nuts and seeds such as almonds, sunflower seeds, macadamias, walnuts, Brazil nuts, avocados, olive oil and fish.

Saturated fats

Saturated fats are OK in moderation, but you don't want to be consuming a large amount. Saturated fats are found in milk, cheese, coconut oil, butter, cream and fattier cuts of meat.

There's been a fad with people talking about how good coconut oil is for you and how you should be using it for everything and just smearing over your food and in your coffee.

This is a big no-no! If you follow this route you could see your LDL (bad cholesterol) skyrocket.

We were never designed to consume large amounts of saturated fats because we just never had access to them. If you flood your body with them, you're setting yourself up for trouble.

Trans fats

These are the fats you want to avoid at all costs. They include: deep-fried foods, baked goods like doughnuts and biscuits, and basically all of the yummy stuff you know is bad for you. These types of fats will wreak havoc on your body and will not set you up for a long and healthy life which is why you should only eat these occasionally.

CHOOSING A COOKING OIL

There has been a lot of research stating that you want to avoid cooking with oils that have low smoke points.

This means that they can't be used at high temperatures. Once these oils reach a certain temperature they become rancid and will cause problems in your body.

If you're going to cook with oil, I suggest using either a small amount of coconut or olive oil. Avoid using plant oils such as sunflower oil or rape-seed (canola oil), soybean, corn, safflower, peanut, etc.

I would also check the label on foods that are "healthy" to make sure that they don't contain these either.

This is because polyunsaturated and monounsaturated fats are highly unstable at high heats. Unless you're getting them from a source like fish or fish oil, then when they're exposed to heat they become oxidised and can cause inflammation in your body and a mutation in your cells.

So, stay clear as much as you can.

Two thumb-sized servings of healthy fats at each meal are going to be your best option.

CARBOHYDRATES (CARBS)

Carbs aren't the devil either and they're essential for muscle building, giving you energy and preventing you from wanting to rip your co-worker's face off when you haven't eaten any in three days.

When it comes to measuring carbs, make a cup with your hands (pictured right) to use as a portion. I suggest only using one hand portion for each normal meal.

If you've just finished a workout then add two cupped handfuls.

If you're trying to gain more muscle and put on weight, have two cupped sized carb servings at every meal.

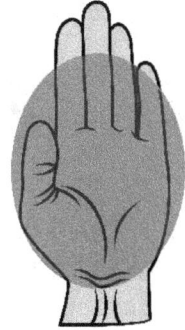

GAINING MUSCLE

If your goal at this time is to gain lean muscle, then you need to be eating more energy than you burn during the day.

A lot of people come to me and ask how they can lose the belly and gain muscle at the same time. The truth is that, unless you're a complete beginner in the gym, this is very hard to do.

The reason for that is because you're trying to give the body too many things to do at once and the body doesn't like change.

It likes to stay exactly where it is comfortable, in a state called "homeostasis". You have to give it a reason to either grow or to lose fat.

When trying to build lean muscle, you should be aiming to gain about 0.25kg (0.5lbs) a week. This way you're optimising the amount of muscle you're gaining and minimising fat gain.

The quicker you put on weight, the more likely you're going to put on fat too because the body can only build so much lean muscle in a certain amount of time.

So if you've got a 12-week goal to build some lean muscle, you should focus on trying to gain about 2-4kg (4-8lbs).

It may not seem like a lot but if your weights are increasing in the gym, you're getting stronger, you're feeling better, you have more energy, and you're slowly looking better, the majority of the weight you've put on will be lean muscle.

LOSING FAT

If your goal is to lose fat, then you need to be eating less food than you burn during the day.

Depending on how heavy you are and how much weight you need to lose, your goal should be to lose no more than one per cent of bodyweight per week.

So, if you weigh 100kg (220lbs) then losing 1kg (2lbs) a week is a pretty good goal to aim for. When you first start reducing your food you may lose more than this and that's because of the amount of water you shed from your body.

Weight loss and weight gain are not always linear either. Even though I've given you some numbers to aim for, it's not going to go as planned.

The scales might tell you that you're on the exact same weight for a week or two and then whoosh it drops 1-2kg and stays at that weight for a few weeks before whooshing again.

We're all different and our bodies can be crazy. We can't choose exactly how it's going to lose weight.

DETERMINING HOW MUCH FOOD YOU NEED

Although you have a guideline to follow above by using your hands, figuring out how much food you're going to need to achieve your goal is determined by a number of factors, such as age, sex, weight, height, body fat, activity level, the types of food you're eating, job, etc.

You're also never going to determine exactly how much you're going to need because of the changes in your life, so what we're looking for is a ballpark number.

While following the guide above and using portion sizes, you should also track your food to see if you're consuming the too little or too much.

There is a free calculator you can use to plug some numbers in and find out how many calories you need based around your goals. You can find it at www.precisionnutrition.com/weight-loss-calculator

Most guys will burn around the 2,400 to 2,600 calories a day on average. If you're eating 2,400 calories and you're not losing or gaining weight, this is called "maintenance".

If your goal is to gain, the first thing to do is to increase the number of calories you're eating by ten per cent

If your goal is to lose fat, then you want to aim to decrease the number of calories you're eating by ten per cent.

Track how much food you're eating during the week to discover exactly how many calories you're taking on board.

Use MyFitnessPal, which is an app that allows you to enter in all of the food you eat for the day and find out how many calories each contains.

The reason tracking calories is so important is that when you have a look at how much you're eating on a weekly basis you're able to see what you need to change.

I'm not expecting you to track all your food for the rest of your life, but having an understanding of how much you're putting into your body is essential in knowing where you are so you can plan where you're going.

Try tracking your food for at least four to eight weeks to see if your portion sizes and calories are matching up using MyFitnessPal.

The type of intermittent fasting approach you plan to follow will determine how much you eat each day.

If you're following Time-Restricted Eating, then you need to be aware that you're eating less than you burn every day.

If you're following Alternate Day Fasting or Whole Day Fasting then you can be more flexible because on the days you're eating considerably less food you're going to be able to put yourself in a deficit quite easily.

BONUS TIP: EATING MORE VEGETABLES

A lot of people struggle to eat enough vegetables. Some give the most ridiculous excuses, such as not liking the taste!

Right, so you're willing to make yourself sick and feel terrible the next day by going out on a Friday or Saturday doing vodka or tequila shots and eating the greasy food at the end of the night, but you won't eat a few greens?

You're willing to drink yourself into oblivion, but you're not willing to give your body the vitamins, minerals and nutrients it needs to improve your health and make you feel amazing?

It's time to take a step back and reconsider what your goals are and how you are taking care of your body.

You're not a child any more. You have to learn to eat loads of vegetables if you want a thriving, healthy body. They provide you with energy and help you stay fuller for longer. They are full of important vitamins and minerals your body needs for things like hormone functions, losing body fat, tissue repair, aiding digestion and giving your body life.

There are hundreds of different types of vegetables out there. You can't use the excuse of not liking the taste because I guarantee there are enough to suit all tastes.

When I talk about vegetables, I'm not just talking about broccoli or green beans. There is cauliflower, eggplant, cucumber, Brussel sprouts, mushrooms, tomatoes, sweet potato, carrot, pumpkin, artichokes, asparagus and so many other different options for you to try.

Set a goal to try one new vegetable every week until you find some that you like and then add them to your diet.

Every night before you go to bed, cut up five handfuls of different types of vegetables, throw them in a container for the next day and you're good to go.

When you buy frozen vegetables, leave some in the freezer at work and some in the freezer at home so you can just pop them in the microwave for a few minutes when you need them.

Every morning when I break my fast with my smoothie I make sure it's chock-full of nutrients and I fill that bad boy up with some vegetables.

Throw in a handful of veg, add in a scoop of protein, one piece of fruit and you've given yourself a bunch of much-needed fibre and nutrients.

Here's a quick example:

- 1 handful of spinach
- 1 stalk of celery
- ¼ beetroot
- ¼ capsicum
- ¼ cucumber
- 1 silver beet leaf
- 1 banana
- 1 scoop of chocolate protein powder

Blend that sucker together and chug it down. The best thing about protein powder and fruit is that it masks the taste of the vegetables, so you won't notice it at all. Don't scrunch up your face thinking that sounds disgusting. Learn to give something a try first before you judge it.

No one (including me) wants to consume something that tastes gross. I want it to taste good and give me the nutrients I need and I expect you will want the same thing.

ISMAEEL RAZAVI – THE GREEN SMOOTHIE KING

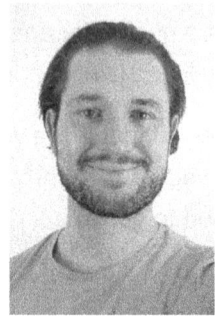

I'm all about starting the morning properly and my daily green smoothie does just that. Apart from instantly feeling amazing, I know that psychologically I'm setting myself up for a healthy and productive day.

I like variety so I opt for spinach, kale, celery, fresh lemon juice, parsley stalks and occasionally add a little apple or pineapple and a touch of honey to sweeten things up!

I swapped my morning coffee for green smoothies and feel so much better for it

---

☑ **TIP:** I've created another ten smoothie recipes for you to download. It's in the resources.

ACTION STEPS

1. Brainstorm how you can turn your "cheat meals" into treat meals. For example: Eating out a nice restaurant instead of McDonald's or eating half a pizza instead of a whole pizza.
2. Write down the days you plan to have your two "treat meals" for the week.
3. Write down some problems that you think will come up while starting intermittent fasting (going out with friends, binge eating, etc.).
4. Write down what you will do when you do make a mistake. For example: "I will get right back on track with my next meal", or "I will eat some food before going out with friends to avoid over-eating."
5. Use your hands for portion sizes.

5
COOKING, SUPPS AND MEAL PREP

Below is a list of all of the best quality carbohydrate, protein and fat sources you can have.

I suggest you print this list out because this will allow you to pick the types of foods you want for the week at the shops.

☑ **TIP:** You can download all of these lists below from the resources section.

PROTEIN	CARBOHYDRATES
• Chicken • Fish • Eggs • Beef • Pork • Tempeh • Tofu • Kangaroo • Goat • Lamb • Protein powder • Greek yoghurt	• Potatoes (any kind) • Oats • Rice (any kind) • Bread (two slices per meal) • Quinoa • Legumes • Fruit • Carrots • Buckwheat

FATS	VEGETABLES
• Avocado	• Artichoke
• Macadamias	• Asparagus
• Pecans	• Broccoli
• Almonds	• Broccolini
• Cashews	• Bok choy
• Pistachios	• Kale
• Walnuts	• Cucumber
• Brazil nut	• Zucchini
• Sunflower seeds	• Peppers
• Flax Seeds	• Pumpkin
• Chia Seeds	• Cauliflower
• Peanut butter	• Tomatoes
• Olive Oil	• Spinach
• Coconut oil	• Mushrooms
• Coconut cream	• Lettuce
• Coconut milk	• Eggplant
• Cashew butter	• Leek
• Eggs	• Any other vegetable you can think of
• Fish oil	
• Milk	
• Cheese	
• Dark chocolate (85% cocoa solids or more)	

SPICES	SAUCES AND CONDIMENTS

• Cinnamon
• Salt
• Pepper
• Chilli
• Mint
• Coriander
• Nutmeg
• Cilantro
• Basil
• Dill
• Turmeric
• Cumin
• Thyme
• Parsley
	• Mustard
	• BBQ or tomato sauce
	  (no sugar options)
	• Low sodium soy sauce
	• Tabasco
	• Apple cider vinegar
	• Normal vinegar
	• Balsamic vinegar
	  (no added sugar)

SUPPLEMENTS

I'm not here to tell you that all these usual supplement brands are crap and then try to sell you my own special package that'll magically help you burn fat.

The truth is you shouldn't even worry about supplements until you get your diet sorted.

If you can't control what you put in your mouth and you keep eating processed food, then supplements aren't going to do anything for you.

Despite saying that, I understand you might still want to look into supplements, so here's my advice.

PROTEIN POWDER

Protein powder won't make you big and it won't make you bulky. If that were the case, there would be a lot more guys and girls walking around looking bigger and with bulging with muscle. (I also wish this was me.)

There's nothing fancy about protein powder and you're far better off getting protein from actual food sources like meat, fish, chicken, etc.

If you're short on time or you're busy all day, that's when I would suggest having protein powder.

I have one scoop of protein in my morning shake because my first "meal" is when I'm training clients and breaking my fast.

Pulling out some chicken or beef to chomp on in the gym is not the best look for a trainer.

If you're looking for a good brand of protein there's only one I use and it's called True Protein. They get their protein from grass-fed cows in New Zealand and it's not loaded with crap. They've also got some great tasting flavours. This is only available in Australia and New Zealand.

If you're outside of Australia and New Zealand, the protein powder you should look for is a simple WPI (whey protein isolate) that is 90 per cent pure protein. I recommend using a brand called Optimum Nutrition, which is the most popular supplement company in the world.

FISH OIL/KRILL OIL

Omega 3s are a must-have in your diet. Brain health, heart health and cell function are all extremely important and you need omega 3s to be performing at your best.

If you're not eating enough fatty fish (trout, salmon, sardines, mackerel etc.) during the week (three times minimum), then you need to be supplementing with an omega 3 supplement daily.

There's a lot of debate about whether to take fish oil or krill oil but if you aren't taking either I suggest you just pick one. It doesn't matter whether you buy it in liquid form or in capsules but if you're going to buy capsules you will have to do the bite test. Bite into a capsule to see if it's fishy tasting. If it is, you need to throw it away because the oil is rancid and bad for you. Fish oil should have NO fishy taste at all.

VITAMIN D

Depending on where you are in the world or if you're sitting in an office all day, there's a good chance you're vitamin D deficient if you hardly go outdoors or go home straight after work.

First off, get your vitamin D levels checked with a blood test. The following recommendation might seem like jibber jabber until you get your results, but then you can compare them to see where you're at.

For optimal health, adults should be aiming for a Vitamin D level of between 120-150 nmol/L. Once there, you can safely take 3,000-4,000 IUs (as a supplement form) a day to maintain healthy Vitamin D levels.

If you are under 100 nmol/L, you can safely take 8,000-10,000 IUs (as a supplement form) to get you up to the optimal range.

If you are obese or elderly, you will most likely need to take 8,000 IUs a day ongoing.

There's a great app called 'D minder'. It is free and it will tell you exactly how much time you need to be spending in the sun every day based on where you're located.

MAGNESIUM

This has worked wonders for my sleep and muscle recovery.

Magnesium powder is the best to buy and take before bed to help your body start relaxing.

One thing I noticed before taking magnesium is that I didn't really dream a lot. This meant I wasn't getting into deep and REM sleep (the best types of sleep). All of that changed once I started using magnesium powder. Not only do I dream every night, but I also feel more relaxed and chilled out before getting into bed.

Magnesium is one of the most common nutrient deficiencies out there and it's probably because people don't eat enough green vegetables. If this sounds like you, you're probably deficient.

Buy yourself some magnesium powder if you feel like you aren't getting enough.

CAFFEINE

No, not pre-workout – just regular black coffee, or green or black tea. All of the "pre-workout fat-burning" supplements out there are just complete BS.

When you look at the main ingredients of many of these fat burners and pre-workouts their main ingredient is caffeine – just a lot more of it per serving than you would usually have.

If you need a pick-me-up before a workout then stick to coffee or tea and save your money to spend on better quality food.

Another problem with people taking pre-workouts is that it disrupts sleep or makes them jittery and anxious.

When this happens, you're now actually preventing yourself from losing fat because you're now not getting enough sleep, which will lead to food cravings during the day, poor energy levels and you will be moving less.

A nice black coffee, green tea or black tea is the only fat burner you need. That being said, if you still want to take pre-workouts then by all means go ahead – just educate yourself beforehand.

CREATINE MONOHYDRATE

Creatine is not essential, but it's one of the only supplements "proven to work".

If you eat a lot of red meat then you're probably getting enough, but if you want to play it safe and supplement you can.

Creatine will help with your strength gains (not by a lot), but you will be able to do an extra rep or two of a given exercise.

Keep in mind that creatine will cause you to store more water. This means you may gain 1-2kg (2-5lbs) in the first few weeks.

Don't stress out if this happens to you and you think you've put on weight. It's just your muscles being able to store more water.

One 5g dose daily is enough and you can mix it in with any drink you choose. I usually add it to my morning smoothie.

Creatine is also extremely cheap and all you need is normal creatine monohydrate. Don't be fooled by websites or supplement companies trying to sell you some "special blend" of creatine.

Does it work for everyone? No. Some people are just non-responders, so you will have to play around with it.

If you eat plenty of red meat, you don't put on any weight when you take it or you don't notice any difference in your strength then you're most likely a non-responder

VITAMINS AND MINERALS

One of the safest bets to see if you need to supplement with anything is to get your blood work done.

A blood test will show you what you're deficient in because there's no point in spending money on supplements when you could be buying better quality food.

If you just want to have a backup and take a multivitamin then the power is yours, but make sure you know what you're taking.

But try to get most of your nutrients from whole, nutritious sources of food and you won't need to worry about taking supplements. Plus, you can use the money you save and spend it on something better.

MEAL PREP

Meal prep is in this book and for a good reason. Just because you're doing intermittent fasting it doesn't mean that you don't have to worry about preparing your meals.

The people who lose weight and manage to keep it off successfully are those who exercise consistently every day and eat the same types of food on a recurring basis.

No, you don't have to eat steamed broccoli and vegetables every day. But during the week you should have a few different food choices you love and that you've prepared ahead so you can rotate through them.

That's also the reason I created that list of the protein, carbs and fat sources that you can choose from. So, when it comes to meal prepping every week, you can create whatever you want and still make sure it's on the right track towards your goals.

Here's what to do when it comes to meal prep:

PICK A TIME

Every week you must pick a time to prepare your meals and I suggest doing this one of two different ways:

1. Do it once a week on a weekend and spend longer in the kitchen preparing the whole week.
2. Do it once on the weekend and once during the middle of the week to split up the time in the kitchen (I do this method).

Once you've picked which suits you best, you then need to book out that time in your calendar to get it done.

Am I serious? Of course I am! How easy is it to skip meal prep if you don't have it booked in? If a friend wants to catch up on a Sunday morning and you forgot that you need to meal prep then you're going to hurt yourself in the long run.

You can avoid that by putting the time in your calendar and set it on a weekly repeat. I make this the first part of my Sunday morning routine before anything else. I go shopping as soon as I'm awake, come back and just do meal prep for the next hour.

Before anyone else in the house is awake I've already finished cooking, got my meals in the fridge and freezer and the rest of the day is mine.

There are two reasons I like doing it in the morning:

1. No one else is awake so there are no distractions and you won't get messaged by a friend that early.
2. No one is at the grocery store, so I'm not mucking around waiting for people and trying to fight my way through the aisles and checkout.

LAY EVERYTHING OUT

Having to go back and forth to the pantry and the fridge to get foods can be a real pain in the ass and ends up taking more time than you thought.

Get all the food and equipment out on the kitchen bench so you have it all there to use. Here's a list of what you will usually use:

- knives
- chopping board
- pots
- pans
- rice cooker

- containers
- cooking oil
- blender
- food
- spare plastic bag to use for scraps
- baking tray and paper

Try to lay it out so you've got some room to breathe but when you have it all in front of you, you know where it all needs to go.

EXPECT IT TO TAKE LONGER THAN YOU THINK

When you first start meal prepping, it's going to take longer than you think. You might be in the kitchen for a few hours until you get used to cooking and doing multiple things at once.

I've now got my meal prep down to one hour on a Sunday using only two stove-top cookers and a tiny mini-oven. If I can prep that quickly with minimal equipment, you should become a pro in no time.

MAKING TIME GO QUICKER

There's nothing more boring than slaving away in a kitchen for a few hours and not having something to listen to. Put on your favourite music, a TV show, or listen to a book or podcast while doing your prep.

DECIDING WHAT TO EAT

One reason most people decide not to do meal prep is they just don't know what to eat. How can you cook for a week if you don't know what to cook?

> ☑ **TIP:** I've got a meal plan template that you can download. It's in the resources.

I want to show you the best way to get started and be able to make your own choices. Let's be honest, some of what you see in the Google results when you look up "meal prep" is pretty bland and ordinary or is unrealistic because it requires a lot of time.

The chart that I listed above is going to be your recipe guide to creating your own meals from the week. It's pretty simple. All you have to do is choose one item from each of the lists and mix them together.

For example:

SOURCE	EXAMPLE
Protein	Kangaroo
Carbs	Sweet potato
Healthy fats	Avocado
Vegetables	Broccoli
Condiment	Chilli sauce

Boom! You've just created yourself an epic lunch for three weekdays.

Now for the next three days, you do the same thing:

SOURCE	EXAMPLE
Protein	Beef mince
Carbs	Kidney beans
Healthy fats	Olive oil
Vegetables	Zucchini, capsicum and canned tomatoes
Condiment	Taco mix

For six days of the week, you've just created two different types of meals you can eat for lunch and dinner.

By making a bulk batch you can save them up and freeze them. The power is yours when it comes to meal prepping and you don't have to rely on anyone else.

When it comes to knowing how much of each food to use that's where the portion sizes of your hands come into play.

Here's a quick reminder:

- Protein – two palm-sized servings
- Carbs – one cupped handful
- Healthy fats – two thumb-sized servings
- Vegetables – two big fists

FREEZING FOOD

You can save yourself a lot of time by freezing food after you've made it, plus it's going to stop it from going off and you having to throw it out. Most food will stay fresh for two to three days depending on what it is. But the last thing you want is to prep your meals for the week and then have them go off.

Freeze your meals for Thursday, Friday and Saturday and keep Monday, Tuesday and Wednesday's in the fridge.

That way on Wednesday night you can take out the other meals and they will be thawed by the morning.

Another great thing about being able to freeze your food is that you can save yourself lots of time by bulk meal-prepping for more than a week.

Let's say you've come up with a few recipes that you really enjoy. For example, the chilli con carne recipe that I share with you in the free plan. Instead of creating it for just a week, why not buy four times the quantity, cook it all (since it will take exactly the same amount of time) and then freeze it for whenever you need it?

You could have a month of several different meals in your freezer just ready to grab and go when you need them and you can change what you feel like.

Maybe tomorrow you'll feel like a chicken stir-fry and remember you've still got a few of them in the freezer.

Preparing meals ahead of time is going to be one of the biggest payoffs for helping you to keep on track, make the right choices and to eat the right types of food.

SHOPPING

Once you know what you want to cook this week, you then need to create a shopping list.

It seems pretty obvious, but there are plenty of times I've gone to the supermarket and forgotten what to buy and then get angry when I come home and realise I've got no carbs for the next couple of meals.

The easiest way to create a shopping list is to use the notes app on your phone to write down exactly what you need. I like to create mini labels depending on where things will be in the store. For example:

FRUIT AND VEGETABLE SECTION	COLD SECTION
• Capsicum • Sweet potato • Apples	• Milk • Chobani Greek yoghurt • Chicken breast

CANNED SECTION	FROZEN SECTION
• Canned tomatoes • Chickpeas • Tuna	• Frozen berries • Frozen fish • Frozen vegetables

HEALTH FOOD SECTION	COOKING SECTION
• Nuts • Bone broth • Health nut butters	• Thyme • Olive oil • Salt and pepper

When you group all of these foods together you're less likely to forget a certain item. You're also not running around the supermarket, going back and forth because you forgot one thing in the veggie aisle and then another thing in the canned aisle.

Write it all down and group it together so you know exactly what you need and where it is.

NAVIGATING THE SUPERMARKET

When you get to the supermarket, you need to have a game plan. There's no point just wandering around, getting distracted and tempted by all of the bad foods that are in there.

Have you ever come home from the store and realised you've just bought 12 bars of chocolate? We want to avoid that.

The golden rule when it comes to navigating the supermarket is to stick to the outside aisles for 90 per cent of your shopping.

The vegetables, the cold section and the frozen section are where most of your shopping should be done.

The only time you're going to go down the middle aisles is when you need to get cans (like tomatoes, sardines and tuna), fermented foods (like sauerkraut) and also your healthy fats like nuts and peanut butter.

Try and avoid the other aisles as much as possible because the more time you spend in them, the more chance you're going to slip up and buy some junk that's on special.

Stick to your shopping list. Go in there with your blinders on, get what you need and get out ASAP.

☑ TIP: Make sure you eat before you go food shopping or go there when you're least hungry. I've made so many mistakes buying what my eyes wanted just because I was starving. Then all of a sudden these "bargains" start to appear and – like I said earlier – 12 packets of chocolate bars fall in the basket.

Being as quick as possible is key when it comes to food shopping and meal prep. The less time you have to spend shopping and prepping, the more time you can go about doing other things you enjoy.

DON'T FORGET CONTAINERS

This part is vital – because once you've prepped all your meals, you're going to need somewhere to store them – so remember to buy yourself plenty of containers.

Again, this might seem simple, but I have made this rookie error a few times. Buy yourself a good set of glass containers that you can use over and over again. They're well worth the investment.

CLEARING THE PANTRY

Another major factor to keep you on track during your weight loss journey is your environment – especially what food is kept at home in the fridge and pantry.

It's easy to slip up and eat something bad if you know it's in the house and is easily accessible.

If you have chocolate in the pantry, it will eventually be eaten. If you've got ice cream in the freezer, it will eventually be eaten.

Maybe not by you, but someone is going to eat it.

The key is to clear out your pantry, your fridge and anywhere else you may keep food to get rid of everything you know is bad for you. This might be hard if, like me, you don't like throwing food away. But this step is crucial.

You may also tell yourself that you don't need to chuck bad stuff out because you have strong willpower or that's not you.

Bullshit!

We're all human and we will give in. Maybe not today, but there will be days.

In order for long-term success, you can't have trigger foods hanging around all the time because there will be days where you're hankering for a snack.

You go searching the pantry or freezer and lo and behold you manage to find a big packet of chips or a litre of ice cream. Then ten minutes later you're standing there with an empty ice cream container and the fridge door open wondering what just happened. You feel extremely guilty and start to hate yourself.

I'm sure most people have been there before. I know I have. Actually, I've been there more than once. When I was younger, it was an occasional thing for me to binge after dinner because I'd be craving something sugary and sweet.

I'd go on the hunt to try and satisfy my cravings and there were times where I would eat an entire cake that was in the fridge all in one go – and then I'd hate myself for the next three days.

SAM – MEAL PREP KING

I dedicate a good time on Sundays to meal prep.

Depending on how busy the Saturday's plans are, I'll usually order my groceries online (it is so easy!). Since they arrive at my door that night, I don't have to spend time doing the shopping and this also keeps me away from temptations.

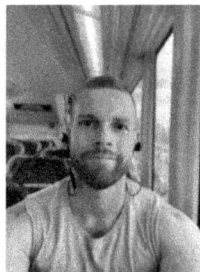

On the Sunday, I switch on my latest favourite bangers on Spotify, and kick everything off with the meat! It's so worth doing as you can get the majority of the prep done in a good 90 minutes, chuck it in the freezer and then you are set for up to two weeks.

Don't bring bad food home with you either.

If you go out for ice cream or you buy an unhealthy snack, make sure you get rid of it before you get home. If it gets into your house it's going to sit there nagging at you, waiting for that time you come in from work after a hard day and you feel lazy, don't want to cook and just want to pig out a little as stress relief.

All of these sneaky foods that you tend to snack on from time to time will wind up adding up to a lot of extra pounds on the scale.

You may do this out of old habits on your first shopping trip while buying your list of foods. You come home and may realise that you slipped up and bought something you shouldn't have.

But since you're throwing away all of the bad stuff, you can quickly get rid of it before it becomes a problem.

And if you don't want to waste the food, give it to your neighbour or bring it in for co-workers. Just don't let the excuses in your head be the reason you don't do this.

FRESH VS FROZEN

You might have the best intentions to eat well, but because you have a busy life and get caught up at work or go out with friends, you find all of those fresh vegetables you bought will start to go off after a few days.

A simple way to stop this is to use frozen veg. You can buy frozen steam bags that you pop in the microwave for a few minutes and – boom – you've got yourself a few servings of vegetables.

The great thing about frozen vegetables is that they're also picked at their peak, which means they're full of nutrients and you're getting all of the good vitamins and minerals.

Spinach is a great veg to buy frozen because you can chuck a few of those frozen blocks in your smoothie in the morning and you're getting a few extra nutrients without even tasting it.

The steam bags are really useful to keep in your freezer at work, because if you forget your lunch one day you will have them to use. You can wander down to the shops to buy a can of tuna or a ¼ piece of rotisserie chicken to go with it.

BONUS TIP: KILLING HUNGER CRAVINGS

Hunger cravings are going to show up when you first start intermittent fasting and there's no real way you can cure them.

The body is going to be hungry because it's used to eating at a certain time, and when you change that time it's going to send a signal to your brain saying: "Hey it's time to eat!"

In order to combat this, drink a lot more liquid first. More water, black coffee, soda water, etc. You're going to pee a lot more at first too, but in order to keep those hunger cravings at bay and not give in to temptation, it's the safest way.

Another suggestion is to eat a meal higher in fat and protein the night before. This takes longer for the body to digest and break down, which means you're not going to be as hungry.

Have a meal that contains either salmon or some avocado and also a lot of vegetables to help increase your fibre intake.

Fat, protein and fibre in food are what help to keep you fuller for longer as it takes the body longer to break down.

During the mornings, just stick to your black coffees and green teas and it won't take long (about two weeks) for the body to adjust to your new eating habits.

PLANNING AHEAD

While I was writing this book, I went to visit my family up in Townsville for the weekend.

My family eat quite healthily, but their fridge is often pretty empty when I go there and doesn't have a lot of vegetables.

The previous time I went, which was more than ten months before, I did some food shopping and decided to try an experiment.

I put some frozen vegetables in the deep freezer outside to see if they would still be there for me next time I came to visit.

When I arrived home that late afternoon I was starving. My family were going to pick up some takeaway for dinner on the way home. I was tempted but I decide to pass and just see what they had in the house.

As soon as I got there I checked the fridge and, lo and behold, it was pretty bare just as I had expected. They had some meat but not any vegetables.

I went to the outside freezer and there were my frozen veg from the time before – still there for when I needed them.

Luckily, I didn't have to give into temptation that night and it was all because I planned ahead of time.

Think about places you frequent, such as work or your partner's house, and just see if you can stock up their freezers with a few packets of frozen foods.

This will save you a lot of headaches and guilt. Planning ahead is preparing to win!

30-DAY RESET

When you first start trying to implement the intermittent fasting diet you need to give yourself a 30-day "reset" to get your body used to this new way of eating and living.

Because your body isn't used to it, it's going to be hard to adapt. But after the 30 days, this way of eating and living is going to be a habit that you can have to for rest of your life.

Thirty days is a drop in the ocean when you compare it to the next ten years of your life. It's best to start it as soon as possible.

You've learned about getting rid of trigger foods, doing your food shopping and meal prep to buy healthy meals for the week. This is the perfect time for you to set yourself up for success.

When it comes to these 30 days you want to focus on eating the best quality food possible, eliminating all of the trigger foods and avoiding alcohol at all costs.

Wait a minute! Didn't I say you can drink alcohol, eat the foods you love and still enjoy yourself without dieting?

Yes, I sure did, but you should eliminate alcohol and trigger foods from your life first to show yourself that you can actually do it and how much better you feel when you do.

Another good reason is because when you do a 30-day reset and eliminate all of the junk food and alcohol from your diet, you're getting a sneak peek at how good you're going to feel and the results you can accomplish by making a few simple changes.

You're going to have a lot more mental clarity, focus and energy.

The only thing you're going to be cutting out is alcohol and processed foods; you can still have your rice and carbs. You can still have your peanut butter, but you're just not having a whole pizza.

After the 30 days you can then apply the 90/10 rule and have ten per cent of your food coming from your "treat food". The first week or two are going to be the hardest because that's when you will experience the cravings. That's when temptations will pop up and your friends are going to try to convince you to throw it all away.

But you need to be tough.

> ☑ **TIP:** You can download your 30-day reset guide from the resources section.

It's more of a guided template as opposed to strict rules, and you'll learn what foods you can swap. For example: if you don't eat red meat but you do eat chicken, you can substitute that.

What you're going to notice is that there is a large quantity of food in this reset phase and there's also a lot of vegetables.

The goal is to show you how you can thrive, eat lots of food and still be able to lose body fat. You shouldn't have to starve in order to lose weight, especially when adopting intermittent fasting approaches.

You should also try out my 2MAD System. I have been trialling a different style of intermittent fasting because I wanted to improve my productivity during the day.

I started only eating twice a day in a six-hour window. I eat my first meal (a nutrient-packed smoothie) at 11am and then a second, bigger meal at 4.30pm.

This gives me a good five-hour window between meals to digest the food, and also stop the distraction of having to cook lunch in the middle of the day when I am at my peak levels of work.

By being able to eliminate that middle of the day chunk of time, I've been able to focus more and get more done. Plus, my energy levels still feel great since the type of foods I put in my smoothie are a nutrient power-house.

Remember: Health and fitness is about thriving, not surviving – so trial-ling different things is key!

> ☑ **TIP:** Plan ahead to decide what you're going to do every week-end, so you don't get distracted by going out for drinks with mates or end up going out for dinner unexpectedly and ruining everything.

Also, hold yourself accountable by making it public on social media. You can join my private group with others on the same journey as you: www.facebook.com/groups/transformingwithtyson

Some other ideas are to:

- eat a good meal before shopping
- create a shopping list
- stick to the outside aisles first and buy all the food you need, shop in the middle aisles last, if at all
- make Tupperware™your friend and buy lots of containers for food prep
- shop as fast as possible

ACTION STEPS

1. Print out the portion control guide and the list of proteins, carbs, fats and condiments to put on your fridge, you can get the list from the resource section.
2. Print out the 30-day reset guide.
3. Create a shopping list (don't forget containers).
4. Throw away everything that you know is a trigger food for you.

PART TWO

EXERCISE

"Take care of your body it's the only place
you have to live"
- Jim Rohn -

6
WEIGHT TRAINING

Anyone can lose weight without exercising. If you burn more calories than you consume during the day, you will lose weight.

The problem with this is that as well as losing fat, you will also lose muscle and bone mass. This will cause your metabolism to slow down and you will end up with that skinny fat look that nobody wants.

You might look OK in a shirt, but you will have the pudgy belly with no muscle mass. You won't be feeling good about yourself because you will still wake up and look in the mirror and have that belly looking back at you.

You will also decrease your bone mineral density and make yourself more prone to injuries and diseases like osteoporosis.

That is why weight training is so important for building a lean body, getting strong bones, reducing your chances of disease and increasing your metabolism.

There are so many different choices out there including CrossFit, yoga, sports, kettlebells and strongman, just to name a few.

I want to share with you my favourite types of weight training and cardio exercises. These are what I'm an expert in and have also been proven to stand the test of time.

Not to say that CrossFit, marathon running, or strongman are bad things. But most of us (including myself) are more likely to get injured if not taught how to do things properly.

There's nothing worse than just kick-starting your fitness journey and having to take a step backwards because you got hurt.

If you're looking to build an overall good-looking body with some muscle mass, then this is going to be perfect for you.

But if you want to become a pro bodybuilder, CrossFit games athlete or marathon runner then you may want to skip this section because you would be better learning from someone with more experience in those speciality sports.

WEIGHT TRAINING

There are so many weight training workouts available that claim to be the best thing. "Six weeks to bigger guns" or "Get a shredded six-pack by doing these core exercises". This is what you will typically see in the magazines.

The truth of the matter is that most of these articles are bullshit marketing aimed at getting you to buy the magazine and follow a workout that a professional bodybuilder or athlete has done (and were more than likely on drugs during the program).

Yes, most of these people are on drugs, but that's another story. There are great documentaries called Prescription Thugs and Icarus that cover the truth about steroids in the sporting world.

But back to weight training. If you want to build a good-looking body, you need to start with a foundation. You can't chisel a lean physique without building a strong foundation first.

In order to do that you need to focus on exercises that are going to put on the most lean muscle. And they should always be in a workout routine because they're proven to be the most effective in getting results in the fastest time possible.

Unless you're injured or there is something preventing you from doing these movements, learn how to do these exercises.

These fundamentals were taught to me by a great mentor named Dan John, and Tony Boutagy, who I mentioned earlier. I have created my own method from what they taught me.

In every program, make sure you cover the following elements:

- squat
- push
- pull
- lunge
- hinge
- twist
- carry

Why these seven movements? It's because they're what humans have always done.

We've had to squat down to sit, pick up heavy things and to carry them over long distances. We have had to push things over our head and pull ourselves up over obstacles.

We've twisted across our body to reach for something and we've lunged over rocks and logs to avoid or chase animals.

We still do these exact movements today when we have to lift a heavy box at work and carry it out to the car or when we need to pull ourselves over a fence when we've locked ourselves out.

But you are also going to be shown the very many variations of the movements.

SQUATS

- goblet squat
- barbell back squat
- front squat
- Zercher squat
- box squat

☑ **TIP:** Start by learning how to do a goblet squat as this will teach you how to squat properly and get low.

HORIZONTAL PUSH MOVEMENTS

- push-ups
- bench press (dumbbell and barbell)
- dumbbell and cable flys

VERTICAL PUSH MOVEMENTS

- overhead press (dumbbell and barbell)
- high Incline press (dumbbell and barbell)
- decline press (dumbbell and barbell)
- side raises
- front raises

HORIZONTAL PULL MOVEMENTS

- bent over row (dumbbell and barbell)
- single arm row
- seated cable row
- chest supported rows

VERTICAL PULL MOVEMENTS

- chin-ups
- pull-ups
- lat pull-downs

HINGE MOVEMENTS

- deadlifts (trap bar, straight bar, kettlebell)
- back extensions
- cable pull through
- kettlebell swings
- good mornings

CARRIES

- farmer's walks
- waiter walks
- sled pushes
- sled pulls
- heavy backpack carries

TWISTING

- Russian twists
- Pallof press (static holds or moving)
- landmine rotations
- wood chops
- static rotation hold

Using these movements as the foundations of your workout will help you to become more balanced, build a nice-looking physique and become stronger.

There are a lot more movements you will learn as you go on, but there's no point in overwhelming you straight from the get-go.

LEARN TO DO THEM CORRECTLY

☑ **TIP:** You can download your workout templates and access all the how to videos in the resource section.

The bench press was the first exercise I did with when I started going to the gym – and I did it wrong for years.

A lot of people get shoulder injuries when they bench press because of the way they flare their elbows or because they lower the bar to the top of their chest instead of the nipples.

You should not be looking at the bar as it comes down to your chest and you shouldn't be squirming around kicking your feet when it gets heavy. This will lead to bad technique and put you at risk of an injury.

Learn how to do it correctly so you can do it again and again for years to come and avoid getting hurt.

You will notice that there are some exercises not in the list that you will see everywhere such as bicep curls, tricep pushdowns, leg extensions, etc. While these are still good exercises to do, they aren't the most time or muscle efficient.

Your goal is to maximise your results in the gym without spending hours on end doing it. You want to get in, get it done and move on.

You can still build biceps, triceps, quads and abs without all of the isolation exercises.

You will build bigger biceps when you're able to do ten bodyweight chin-ups in a row. You will build bigger triceps when you're able to conquer ten bodyweight dips. You will build a stronger core when you can pick heavy weights off the ground.

Think about this – if you weigh 70kg (155lbs) and you do ten chin-ups, you've just moved 700kg (1,550lbs) with your biceps and back muscles.

Want to try to curl 70kg with ten reps? Not going to happen.

If you can lift more weight more with a given exercise, then you're going to stimulate more muscle growth and get results faster.

Another good reason for lifting heavier weights and doing full body exercises is that you burn more calories doing a squat than you would just doing leg extensions or tricep pushdowns.

This means you're getting the best of both worlds in terms of building muscle and burning more calories.

If you've never been in a gym or don't have experience doing these exercises correctly, hire a personal trainer for a few months to teach you these fundamentals.

Be upfront with them. Tell them that you have a specific list of exercises that you want to learn and don't let them sweet talk you into doing a "special" exercise or a learning a different way.

You're looking to get the best bang for your buck and the simple, most basic exercises have been proven to work the best.

HOW MANY DAYS SHOULD YOU TRAIN WITH WEIGHTS?

Many people make the mistake of not working out enough. Yeah, you read that right.

People will go to the gym a few times a week but aren't training enough as they focus on one body part like the professional bodybuilders.

Have you ever wondered why we train like that? It's probably because we've seen all of the professionals do it, right?

But you are not a professional bodybuilder and are unlikely to be able to dedicate long periods of your day to training. Sometimes you aren't able to go to the gym every day.

Those guys who weigh more than 100kg (220lbs), go in and annihilate one body part and make it sore for seven days before they can train it again are able to get to the gym for several hours every day.

Going back to what I mentioned earlier: Are you on drugs? Are you looking to be a professional bodybuilder? Do you already have 16-inch arms?

If your answer is 'no' to those questions, then you don't need to train like they do.

Next time you're in the gym, have a look around at how guys are following what the so-called experts are doing but still don't look anything like them. Why is that? It's because they didn't build their foundation first.

In order for you to train "enough", you have to be training each body part two to three times per week to stimulate muscle growth.

Studies have shown that after 48 hours of training a muscle, it is fully recovered and able to be trained again.

So if you trained your chest on Monday, you could train it again on Wednesday. But if you're someone who only trains their chest once a week, you're missing out on a lot of muscle gain.

Think about someone who trains their legs every Monday, Wednesday and Friday versus someone who only trains legs only once a week.

If you compared them in a year's time, who do you think will have made more progress both in terms of strength and muscle?

HOW SHOULD YOU WORK OUT?

There are two ways that you can structure your workout and it all depends on how much time you've got.

If you have more free time during the week, then doing four weight training days a week will be best for you. This could be a combination of upper and lower body workouts or pushing and pulling movements depending on your preference.

If you're more time-restricted and can't go as often, then doing a full body routine two to three times a week is more optimal.

The difference between doing a four-day weight training program and a three-day one is the time it takes in the gym.

A lot of people complain about full body workouts because even though they're effective, they can take a long time to complete.

For some people it can take up to 90 minutes and it just becomes a burden. Trying to spend that long in the gym a few times a week for many is simply unrealistic.

The reason people take so long doing full body sessions is that they feel like they have to target every muscle individually and do numerous exercises, but this doesn't have to be the case.

The compound movements listed above target several muscle groups at a time, meaning you can do one exercise instead of three.

Let's take the bench press for example. When you bench press, you're not only working your chest muscles but also your triceps and shoulders. This means that after you've finished the bench press you don't have to do tricep pushdowns or isolation work for your shoulders because you've already used the muscles.

The same goes for a squat.

In a squat you're using your quads, hamstrings, glutes, adductors, abductors, calf muscles and your abs. This is why people talk about the squat being such a good exercise – it's because you're getting a lot of return on your effort.

Don't be fooled about abs training either. If you're getting stronger in the squat, deadlift and other compound movements then your abs are getting worked. Even though you're not "feeling the burn" your abs are still working hard to keep you upright while squatting with a weight on your back, picking something heavy off the ground and pushing something heavy over your head.

FULL BODY WORKOUT

Here's an example of what a routine could look like:

WORKOUT ONE

MOVEMENT	EXERCISE	REPS	SETS
Squat	Back squat	8	4
Push	Bench press	10	3
Pull	Chin-up	10	3
Hinge	Kettlebell swing	10	3
Lunge	Walking lunges	10	3
Twist	Pallof press	10	3
Carry	Farmer's walk	30 secs	3
Hinge	Trap-bar deadlift	8	4
Push	Overhead press	10	3
Pull	Bent-over row	10	3
Squat	Goblet squat	10	3
Lunge	Step ups	10	3
Twist	Static hold	10	3
Carry	Sled push	40 feet	3

Repeat those workouts, alternating them every second day, three times a week. For example:

WEEK ONE

DAY	ACTIVITY
Monday	Workout 1
Tuesday	LISS
Wednesday	Workout 2
Thursday	HIIT
Friday	Workout 1
Saturday	LISS
Sunday	Rest

If you repeat the rotation every two weeks, you can guarantee that every muscle in your body is going to grow and you will not be spending hours in the gym.

FOUR-DAY ROUTINE

If you want to train with weights four days a week then you've got two options as to how you can split your training up.

You can do two upper and two lower body workouts or you can do a two push and two pull workouts. Here's what an example of what those workouts would look like:

SCHEDULE

DAY	ACTIVITY
Monday	Push or upper body
Tuesday	Pull or lower body
Wednesday	LIIS
Thursday	Push or upper body
Friday	Pull or lower body
Saturday	HIIT
Sunday	Rest

PUSH

MOVEMENT	EXERCISE	REPS	SETS
Push	Barbell squat	8	4
Push	Bench press	10	3
Push	Overhead press	10	3
Push/ Lunge	Walking lunges	10	3
Twist	Pallof press	10	3
Carry	Sled push	40 feet	3

PULL

MOVEMENT	EXERCISE	REPS	SETS
Pull	Trap-bar deadlift	8	4
Pull	Chin-ups	10	3
Pull	Bent over row	10	3
Hinge	Back extensions	10	3
Twist	Static hold	30 secs	3
Carry	Farmer's walks	40 feet	3

UPPER

MOVEMENT	EXERCISE	REPS	SETS
Push	Barbell bench press	10	3
Pull	Bent-over row	10	3
Push	Overhead press	10	3
Pull	Chin-ups	10	3
Twist	Static hold	30 secs	3
Carry	Farmer's walk	40 feet	3

LOWER

MOVEMENT	EXERCISE	REPS	SETS
Hinge	Deadlift	8	4
Squat	Goblet squat	10	3
Lunge	Walking lunges	10	3
Hinge	Back extensions	10	3
Twist	Pallof press	10	3
Carry	Sled pushes	40 feet	3

But remember – don't try to force what you can't do. If you want to do a four-day routine, but you only find yourself making it twice a week then you're robbing yourself of gaining muscle, especially if you're following a program that's designed for someone who can come in four days a week.

> ☑ TIP: You can download your workout templates and access all the 'how to' videos in the resource section.

INJURIES

If you're carrying an injury then there will obviously be some exercises you can't do, but you can substitute them for others or change the way you approach it.

For example, if you can't do a barbell bench press because of a shoulder injury then you could swap in something like dumbbells instead. You could also raise the bench on a slight incline or change your hand position from pronated to neutral.

Likewise, if you can't squat because of a mobility issue but you can leg press or do leg extensions, there's nothing wrong with that either.

Everyone is different, and you have to work with the hand you've been dealt. If you try an exercise and it starts causing a sharp pain, numbness, tingling or stinging, then stop.

Don't try to push through it; go and see a physiotherapist to get it checked out. One of the worst things you can do is persist and keep pushing and then cause yourself a bad injury.

Remember not to go too heavy at first either. Learning the correct technique, as I have said, is crucial and lifting too heavy too quickly and allowing your technique to breakdown is not good.

You see guys who squat down halfway, deadlift with a rounded back or bench press by bouncing the bar off their chest, flailing their legs everywhere and their body is squirming (this was me).

Check your ego at the door and always make sure you're practising good form above anything else. If you're trying to go up in weight and you're sacrificing technique, then you're setting yourself up for a world of pain in the future.

PROGRESSIVE OVERLOAD

Each time you go to the gym you should be making some type of progress in order to make your body adapt and grow.

You do this by increasing the amount of weight you use, increasing the number of reps/sets you do, or increasing the intensity.

A complete beginner should start by trying to increase the amount of weight. Each time you go to the gym that week you should aim to lift a little bit heavier.

If you could bench press 60kg (135lbs) for ten reps last week then your goal should be to increase the weight by the smallest increment possible, which will usually be 2.5kg (5lbs). In this case, you would want to try and bench 62.5kg for ten reps.

Is that small of a weight jump really going to help your body build muscle? Absolutely, and it's because your body has never been exposed to it before and you've just lifted 2.5kg more than you've done before.

Those who have been training for a few years should try to increase one of the three overload methods. Even if it's just one or two reps extra, a personal best is a personal best.

You're not going to be able to get a personal best on every single exercise every single time. And life is going to get in the way, stress is going to come up and things will just happen that hold you back, so don't beat yourself up.

Some weeks it's going to be difficult just making it to the gym. But remember that your goal should be trying to make progressive overload happen. It may not always happen but *try* to make it happen.

Every time you come into the gym you need to aim to be improving in one of three ways:

VOLUME

This is the total amount of work done in the session and how much weight you've moved. If you start by squatting 100kg for ten reps for three sets then your total volume is 3,000kg (7,500lbs).

In order to increase your volume, you can increase the number of reps you are doing (moving from ten to 11, for example), increase the number of sets (moving from three to four) or increasing the amount of weight you lifted (100kg to 102.5kg).

The more volume you're able to achieve, the more muscle you're going to build because you're going to be giving your body a new stimulus to adapt to each time it's in the gym.

But when it comes to volume, you don't need to go crazy and increase it by large amounts. There's only so much you can do in the time you have. Increasing volume by adding more reps and more sets means you're going to spend more time in the gym and if you don't have the time then that's going to be a problem.

Increasing volume can be as simple as adding one extra rep each week you come in.

So, if you're doing three sets of ten this week, come in and do three sets of 11 with the same weight next time.

Yes, it's really that simple and your body will grow.

If you're in the beginning phase of training (your first year) then you've got a lot of potential to build the best foundation of muscle if you do it right. Adding just that little bit of extra volume is going to help you gain muscle faster.

INTENSITY

This is just how hard you feel the session is. You can increase your intensity by shortening your rest time. Instead of your usual two-minute rest, cut it down to 90 seconds or one minute to make you work harder with less recovery.

You could also change the intensity by lowering a weight slower and raising it slower than you usually would which would cause the lighter weights to "feel heavier" and increase your intensity.

I'm not a big fan of this method unless you're on a tight schedule. You will make more muscle and strength gains if you take more time to recover between your sets because you will be able to use more weight and do more reps.

STRENGTH

Stronger muscles are bigger muscles and bigger muscles are stronger muscles. One way to get better muscular results is to get stronger. The more weight you can lift, the bigger the muscle will grow.

Always aim to increase the weight on an exercise whenever you can. But keep in mind some exercises will be easier to make progress on than others.

For example, you will be able to increase your weights on squats a lot faster than you can on a bicep curl. One of the reasons for this is just because of the amount of muscles you use. A squat is a whole body movement and requires a lot more muscles than a bicep curl, meaning all of the muscles you use to squat will help you move more weight.

You should aim to increase your weights on the bigger full-body movements every week until it just becomes too hard.

Once you become more experienced, increasing the weight is going to become harder and harder. This is natural.

Your progress will slow down and maybe you will only be able to add weight to the bar every few weeks. This is when you can aim to start increasing the reps instead.

If you look at advanced people who've been training for a long time their progress is even slower and they can be stuck on the same weight for months on end.

Everyone has a different genetic makeup, so I can't say how much strength you will gain in what timeframe, but you need to up the ante whenever you can.

The small changes you add in the gym each time you work out will add up to a lot more muscle growth. That means you will make a lot more progress in the gym than the guys you see day in, day out doing the exact same amount of reps for the exact same sets, with the exact same weight and wondering why their body isn't changing.

MAKING PROGRESS THE SMART WAY WITH PETER MACLEAN

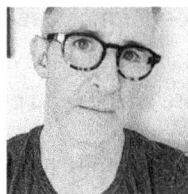

I started training with Tyson in December 2016. I had tried the gym, Pilates and yoga on and off over the years but nothing had stuck. I'd allowed life – meaning work – to get in the way. I was 51 and 88 kilos (15 kilos heavier than I thought I should be).

I was exercising but after six months it was still pretty much, guesswork. At first, it was mainly cardio as my previous knee, hip and ankle problems stopped because I was running lighter. The weights upstairs still held too many unknowns, and a long history of back problems meant I wasn't going to wing it there.

But I was doing something right. I dropped 16 kilos in five months, though maybe as much muscle as fat.

I put together a program from YouTube videos, always running each new exercise past my longstanding physio. Nevertheless, I was missing a solid plan.

At the train station one morning I recognised Tyson as a trainer from the gym. We chatted about nutrition and, having thought about signing up for nutrition advice, I decided to sign up with him as my personal trainer.

It was the single best decision I've made in years.

From the start, the changes have been rapid. My focus shifted from weight loss to a raft of gains. Muscle, strength, definition and – most importantly for someone with a dodgy back from decades sitting at a computer screen – developing a core. And there is the accountability, always the accountability!

ACTION STEPS

1. Download the free workout program from the resource section.
2. Decide how many days realistically you can train with weights every week.
3. Buy yourself a workout planner or download an app you can use to track your workouts.
4. If you don't know how to do any of the exercises, watch the videos on YouTube or hire a trainer.

7
CARDIO

Cardio is crucial for your overall health but there has been some back-lash in the last few years. There are a lot of people who say they don't do any cardio and still manage to lose weight.

That may be all well and dandy, but if you want to live a healthier lifestyle then I don't see why you wouldn't want to include cardio in your workout regime.

We're always trying to chase the "best" cardio workout or ask what's better – treadmill, rower or bike? The answer is that there isn't one best tool that's going to fit everyone.

But there are many options to choose from. Bike riding, jogging, rowing, kayaking, swimming, cross trainer, elliptical, trail walking and circuit workouts just to name a few. I could go on and on, but you get the point. Not everyone loves running; not everyone can run. So, if you don't want to run, you don't have to.

Just pick a few things that you do like doing; things that get your heart rate going and that you can do over and over again but do not feel like a chore.

If you have to force yourself to do 40 to 60 minutes of exercise and dread it every time you come in, then there's very little chance that you're going to stick to it for the long term.

And what you like now may change in the future and that's OK. Just because you love to run doesn't mean you're going to love running in a year from now. You might find another sport that's more fun.

Once you've decided on a few types of exercises that you wouldn't mind doing, you've now got to decide what type of cardio to do.

There are two main sources of cardio to choose from, which are LISS (low intensity steady state) and HIIT (high intensity interval training).

I'm sure you've seen the hype around HIIT training and all the calories you burn. While HIIT is a great tool, it's not the be all and end all. To be honest, you've probably not been getting all of the benefits from HIIT workouts with just ten minutes a day – it takes a lot longer than that to get the most out of it.

Let's look at the different types of cardio in more detail.

LOW INTENSITY STEADY STATE CARDIO

Low intensity steady state (LISS) is something you can do that requires about a three to a six on the effort scale. It's that Sunday morning brisk walk, riding across the city or walking on a trail. It's slightly tough, but it's not killing you.

After 40 to 60 minutes, you should have worked up some type of sweat because this isn't just a leisurely walk.

LISS is great for overall heart health and can be done day in and day out. It's perfect for when you're feeling sore or you just need to burn some extra calories. LISS workouts can be done anywhere depending on what you do, but most people tend to do it in the gym.

The problem with most LISS training in the gym is that it's still boring if you're on the treadmill walking on an incline/light jogging, or you're on a stationary bike. Time can go pretty slow, so here are a few tricks to beat off the boredom:

WATCH NETFLIX

Seriously, Netflix can be streamed to your phone or your tablet and if you just want to come in and zone out for a few hours then I suggest you download a few episodes of your TV series and just go to town.

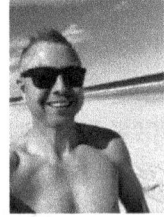

MEET STEVEN, HE'S A NETFLIX MASTER

I usually begin my gym session by walking on a treadmill, using a bike or a cross-trainer while watching an episode of one of my favourite shows on Netflix. It's a great way for me to bump up my step count for the day, burn some extra calories and warm up before I see Tyson for a PT session.

Watching Netflix helps to make cardio just a little bit easier.

Doing this on a regular basis, combined with weight training, has helped me to lose some unwanted fat and get back to the weight I was in high school.

READ A BOOK

I often put the treadmill on a high incline and bump it up to a fast-paced walk – just enough that I can feel I'm working hard, but not hard enough that I can't concentrate – and then I read.

I read more than 52 books a year (including textbooks) and most of them have been while burning some extra calories.

> ☑ **TIP:** Take it slow at first. I don't want people telling me they broke their ankle because they tried to jog while reading a book and fell over.

LISTEN TO BOOKS OR PODCASTS

If you don't want to read a book while exercising and you don't like watching TV, then you can listen to an audio book or a podcast.

You can get lost in a fiction book while listening to it on Audible (a great way to consume books). Or you can just put on some music and pump up the beats.

HIIT TRAINING

HIIT training is all the rage at the moment and it's one of my favourite types of exercises.

Those who like HIIT training are more the type-A people. They're hard-charging, always want to feel like they've killed themselves after a workout and want to feel they have given it their all. HIIT training means you're pushing yourself to a nine or ten out of ten.

If you do HIIT right, you won't want to do it for another few days because it's extremely tough. That's what true HIIT training is.

Doing circuit training with weights for 30 seconds on and 30 seconds rest isn't enough to get your heart rate high enough.

HIIT training is most effective by doing real cardio. Hill sprints, bike intervals, flat sprints, swimming sprints and the likes of these are going to give you the best workout.

These need to be an all-out effort followed by a certain time of rest before going as hard as possible again.

There are a lot of methods you can choose for HIIT workouts and you can apply the same method to any exercise whether it be sprints, bike intervals or swimming, etc.

Here are some examples:

HARD	EASY
1 minute	1 minute
20 seconds	40 seconds
30 seconds	30 seconds
2 minutes	2 minutes
4 minutes	4 minutes
20 seconds	10 seconds
30 seconds	2 minutes

☑ **TIP:** You can download examples and templates of these routines in the resource section.

Use an app called Interval Timer or set the clock on your phone to go off every minute so you don't lose track of where you're at.

SEMI-INTENSITY INTERVAL TRAINING (SIIT)

Semi-intensity interval training is like a mixture of HIIT and LISS workouts. The reason it's a mixture is that you don't go to full 100 per cent exertion on the exercise.

This is a type of training is known as Fartlek or "speed play". It involves you changing your exercise speed. For example, you would go from walking to jogging, to a run and then an all-out sprinting. These changes in tempo speeds are put into intervals.

This allows for maximal efforts without burning yourself out too quickly. It can be done outside, inside, in a pool, or even on a bike. There's virtually no limit on how you can experience the many Fartlek training advantages available to you.

And the great thing about the variety is you can always change from one thing to another and keep your mind guessing!

Here's an example:

INTENSITY	TIME
Medium	8 minutes
Fast	4 minutes
Sprint	20 seconds
Slow	1 minute
Sprint	30 seconds
Slow	1 minute
Sprint	10 seconds
Medium	2 minutes
Sprint	20 seconds
Slow	1 minute
Medium	5 minutes
Sprint	1 minute

COMPLEXES

A complex is a circuit using one piece of equipment, one load, and one space. You load up a bar with a light enough weight that you can complete for every exercise without having to stop.

Perform each exercise one after another until all exercises are completed. Then put the bar down and rest for 90 seconds.

EXERCISE	REPS
Deadlift	8
Romanian deadlift	8
Bent-over row	8
Reverse lunges	8
Front squats	8
Push press	8
Back squats	8
Good mornings	8

As you can see, you go from one thing to another without fully burning yourself out. This is a great style of training to start with to prepare for a true HIIT session.

CIRCUIT TRAINING

Circuit training is a bit different to barbell complexes because you're able to move around more and change to different types of equipment and movements.

It is becoming trendier in gyms and will typically be called an HIIT class or athletic class, when in reality they're just circuit training.

If you've seen the F45 gyms that are blowing up everywhere, this is all circuit-type work. You go from one piece of equipment or exercise to the next with a short break period.

You spend 45 seconds on each station followed by a 15-second rest. Here's an example:

EXERCISE	DURATION (SECONDS)
Burpees	45
Curl to press	45
Treadmill sprint	45
Box jumps	45
Medicine ball slams	45
Jumping lunges	45
Push-ups	45
Russian twists	45
Mountain climbers	45
Trx rows	45

These types of workouts can be extremely tough, especially when you're diligent with your short rest periods.

But don't do this style of training or complexes if you haven't done a lot of explosive-type exercises before as you could risk injury if you're not prepared for it or don't have good form.

BODYWEIGHT TRAINING

If you don't have access to a gym at the moment and you still want to incorporate some type of workout routine into your life, then you can follow a simple bodyweight schedule at home.

The only problem with bodyweight workouts is that there's a limit to what you can do. Eventually you will plateau because you won't be able to continually progressively overload your muscles.

But bodyweight exercises are still a great place to start as they help you become more aware of your body and how to use it.

A lot of people don't have mind/body awareness and can't control certain movements or feel certain muscles working properly.

So being able to take some time to understand how your body moves and why it moves the way it does can help with your progression when it's time for you to step into the gym if you choose to do so.

When doing bodyweight training at home, pick up a few tools to give yourself an even better workout and progressively load your muscles and get more done.

When starting off all you're going to need is a chair and a table. This is important for two reasons:

1. Learning how to squat correctly.
2. Having some type of pulling movement in your workout.

One thing most bodyweight routines lack in is having a pulling movement and it's hard to do that when you don't have a barbell, dumbbell or one of those pull-up bars you can buy.

If you don't have any of those things, then a table will have to do in the meantime.

Once you're able to sit back in a chair and understand what squatting feels like, you'll be able to remove the chair over time and understand what you need to do in order to squat properly.

When you're able to slide yourself to the edge of the table and pull yourself up, you'll be able to get a better workout for your back and biceps and make sure everything is balanced instead of doing too many pressing movements.

If you work from home, you can also do bodyweight exercises during the day to break up your work hours.

You could set a timer on your phone to go off every 50 minutes and for the last ten minutes of every hour you can do a quick circuit workout.

Working this way, you're not stuck behind your desk all day getting the negative effects of long-term sitting. Instead, you're actually doing something positive for your body.

Whether you're doing workouts every ten minutes on the hour or doing 30 to 40 minutes, bodyweight circuits are the best approach as you can get a lot done in a short amount of time.

Here's an example:

- squats
- push-ups
- alternating lunges
- sit-ups
- burpees
- table rows

You would do 15 reps of each exercise and repeat over and over again.

> ☑ TIP: You can download examples and templates of these routines in the resource section.

You will build up your fitness pretty quickly with bodyweight training, which means you will have to find a way to progressively overload your muscles.

A set of dumbbells, a kettlebell and a skipping rope can help you go a lot further with your training than just bodyweight alone.

Kettlebells are excellent because they're versatile and allow you to add so many more exercises into your home workout routine with one piece of equipment.

Buy either two 12kg kettlebells or one 16/20kg kettlebell. You need to get one that's heavy enough to squat, deadlift and swing with, but not so heavy that you can't put it over the head.

Dumbbells are another great piece of equipment to buy because you can use them for so many different activities. And they can be a little bit more challenging, especially if you're able to add and remove weights.

If you're going to get some, buy ones that allow you to strip weights on and off easily to make it heavier and lighter.

SKIPPING ROPE

Who needs running when you can use a rope? I used to do a lot of skipping but it's been a while since I've picked a rope up.

One of my clients, Peter, loves doing intervals on the rope especially when he can't get to the gym and he wants to have some fun. He will just pull out his rope walk into his courtyard and go hard for 20 minutes.

You will see that you don't need much when it comes to home workout equipment but picking up the items suggested will work wonders. It will also allow you to use them for pressing and rows too.

ACTION STEPS

1. Download the free cardio routines and workout routines from the resource page.
2. Pick a few types of exercises that you like.
3. Download a Netflix series you can watch while doing LISS cardio to stop it becoming boring.

8
NEAT TRICKS, SNEAKY STRETCHING & MOBILITY

Maintaining your mobility and stretching regularly are extremely important, especially for people who work in an office all day and are hunched over a computer.

If you can't raise your hands above your head and keep them straight, or you are always waking up and feeling tight, having lower back pain and neck pain, then you need to be working on your mobility.

I'm going to put this out there and admit I don't do this as much as I should – probably like 99 per cent of people – but it doesn't make it any less important.

Most of the pain you're experiencing is probably coming from your short hip flexors, glutes and thoracic areas because they are where most problems tend to happen due to working at a desk.

Long periods of standing are not the answer either. I stand at my desk for most of the day when I'm not training clients. If I'm not paying attention to stretching out my muscles, it really puts a strain on my lower back.

We just aren't meant to sit or stand in one spot for long periods of time. It's not in our DNA. It's killing us slowly and causing all sorts of pain.

If you're incredibly busy and don't think you have time to dedicate to stretching and doing mobility exercises every day, there's a solution for you. Whenever you have a few minutes free while watching TV at home or just sitting around doing nothing, this is the perfect time to do some stretching and foam rolling.

If you're watching your favourite TV show (Game Of Thrones is on as I write this) then you have a whole hour to be moving around on a foam roller and doing some stretching to undo all of the cobwebs that have been building up over time.

You don't have to do much while holding a stretch. You can be in a couch stretch or pigeon pose while watching Jon Snow kill a white walker.

I have a standing desk and at different times throughout the day (usually every 20 to 30 minutes), I'll jump into a different position. I'll put my leg on the desk and stretch out my hip flexor, stand in a tall kneeling position or put my back leg on a chair to stretch my quad.

When you add in these sneaky stretches to improve your mobility and flexibility, you're more likely to stick to it because it doesn't take a lot of effort.

Foam rollers are amazing because they make you feel like a new person when you use them correctly. There's a great book called Deskbound by Kelly Starrett, which teaches how to undo all of the negative stuff you do to your body while working at a desk.

Another great tip is to set a timer on your computer or phone for every 45 to 50 minutes and get up from your desk and walk around the office to get your body moving.

Just doing something as simple as that can help towards undoing those issues.

DO IT IN YOUR DOWNTIME

Taking time to do a five-minute, pre-bedtime routine where you stretch or lay across a foam roller is another excellent way to fit in those mobility exercises. This will also help to calm you down and relax your body so that you're able to get to sleep faster and have a better quality sleep.

Next time you're stretching, just remember how good you feel when you're all limbered up and have cleared the cobwebs.

NON-EXERCISE ACTIVITY THERMOGENESIS (NEAT)

Conventional wisdom makes us think the effort we put into working out will determine whether or not we lose body fat. But exercise is only a small blip on the radar for losing fat.

When you think about it, you're exercising for an hour a day (if you're lucky), which is only a small percentage of time. And there's only so much effort you can put in during that period.

If you do a HIIT workout you might burn anywhere from 200 to 800 calories depending on how heavy you are and your experience level, but that's not a lot in the grand scheme of things.

What if I told you that you could lose more body fat by not slugging it out in the gym for hours on end?

Firstly, if you're like most people, you don't have hours spare to spend in the gym every day doing long cardio sessions. Even if you do have that much downtime, I don't think you want to be spending it all in the gym anyway, unless it's to get away from your spouse (I'm half kidding).

We all have better things to do with our time. So, while putting in a hard effort at the gym is important, there's something you should focus on more because it will get you better results.

Non-exercise activity thermogenesis (NEAT) takes in all of the stuff you do when you're not in the gym such as walking the dog, running for the bus, getting groovy with a partner and everything else you do on a daily basis.

What you don't realise is that NEAT activity can add up over time and have a much greater effect on your weight loss than the amount of time you spend in the gym.

If you sleep for seven hours and spend one hour in the gym, that's eight hours of your day gone. You then have 16 hours of NEAT activity you could be doing during the day that will help burn a lot of extra calories and make your fat loss journey just that little bit easier.

Here are some top tips for NEAT activities to do every day.

MORNING WALKS

Start your day off with a 20 to 30-minute power walk on an empty stomach. Not only is this going to kick-start your metabolism, but because you're doing it on an empty stomach you're going to be burning fat as a fuel source as opposed to carbohydrates.

This will teach your body to become metabolically flexible and switch from fats to carbs when it needs to. It is a morning walk, but make sure you give it some intensity.

Chuck in some headphones and listen to a podcast or audiobook while power-walking outside.

Another great idea is to go to a gym and do an incline walk on the treadmill, or if you have a treadmill at home get it out and do it there.

WALK OR RIDE A BIKE TO WORK

Here in Sydney, it's faster to ride your bike than to drive or take public transport because it's just so busy. I can be at my job in five minutes when I ride my bike but driving easily takes ten to 15 minutes. If you're in a busy city and the traffic is hectic, you can ride past everyone stuck in the jams while you have a massive grin on your face.

FIVE-MINUTE BREAKS

Busy at work? Set a timer for every 30 to 40 minutes and have a five-minute break to get up and go for a walk around the office. Do some bodyweight squats either at your desk or in the bathroom if you care what people will think. Just get moving. If you're at work for eight hours and you go for a five-minute walk every hour that's an extra 40 minutes of activity you've just managed to rack up.

WALK TO GET YOUR GROCERIES

I do my meal prep every Sunday and I walk down to the shops, which are about 15 minutes away, do my grocery shopping and carry it all back in my backpack and green bags (don't use plastic because they're a bitch if they break on the way home).

When you're carrying all of those heavy groceries for the week you notice it gets quite hard walking with all of that stuff and you might even break a sweat.

STANDING DESK

Standing up will help you burn more calories than sitting down. But it's not just the standing; it's also the fidgeting you will do while you're standing up.

You'll notice that you will never just stand still in one place. You'll change your stance, hop side to side and you're more motivated to walk over and speak to your colleague instead of sending them an email.

WALKING AT LUNCH

If you've got an hour lunch, spend 20 minutes eating and the other 30 to 40 minutes going for a walk and getting some vitamin D.

Most people who are stuck in their office all day are also vitamin D deficient. So, while you're outside burning some extra calories, you're also getting your daily dose of vitamin D.

Another great thing about walking after a meal is that it helps with your digestion. Because you've just eaten and now you're standing up and moving, you're increasing blood flow to the gut and not compressing your organs.

WALK TO THE NEXT BUS STOP

If you're waiting for the train or the bus and it's not going to arrive for 15 minutes or so, why not walk to the next stop? It's usually only about ten minutes away so you shouldn't miss it and instead of sitting on your butt doing nothing, you burn some calories.

TAKE THE STAIRS

It is amazing how many people will take the elevator or escalator instead of the stairs. Whenever you get the opportunity, walk up and down the stairs.

WEAR A WEIGHTED VEST

This was suggested on a podcast. I thought it was such a great idea.

This guy wears a 5kg (12lbs) vest wherever he goes. He does his shopping in it, wears it to the gym and even goes to work in it sometimes.

Carrying around an extra 5kg will add up to a lot more calories burned.

You can buy weighted vests that fit snugly under a suit, so it doesn't look like you're wearing a huge jacket.

If you don't want to wear a weighted vest, you could simply add some weight to your backpack or suitcase (think about putting in some big books or heavy items you have around the house).

WALK AFTER EVERY MEAL

Sneaking in an extra ten minutes of walking after breakfast, lunch and dinner will mean 30 more minutes of activity.

Every time I finish eating, I get up and go for a walk to help with digestion. It also gets me away from food, because sometimes I crave a little bit more. But if you get up and leave the kitchen to go for a walk, then you're not going to have it.

CARDIO OR WEIGHTS

People often ask whether cardio or weight training is better for losing stubborn fat. My answer has changed over time.

When I get asked that question now, I always answer with another question first and ask: "Why do you have to choose? You're not bound to only being able to use weights or only being able to use cardio so why are you so concerned about it?"

That answer is usually met with a stony face, so I go on to explain that I would always choose resistance training first. This is because you get a lot of long-term benefits from weight training that will help you build more muscle and burn more body fat.

When you're able to build more muscle with resistance training, you're able to increase the number of calories you burn during the day, and this helps you to burn more body fat.

The problem with just doing cardio and not weight training is that you will lose weight but also your metabolism actually slows down and if you're not eating enough protein you could actually lose muscle too.

So, when in doubt, always aim to start doing your resistance training first if you only have one option for the day.

But it's unlikely you're only going to be able to do just one, and a combination will get you the best results long term. There are so many benefits you get from a combination of both of these styles of training.

What are you in a rush for anyway? Who're you trying to impress? You've got years and years ahead of you to make progress and you want to make them as fun and as pain-free as possible. You're in the gym to build up your body not to break it down and get hurt.

Pain, no gain.

That last bit wasn't me looking down on you and getting all righteous, I actually wrote it to remind myself of the journey. I was always someone in a rush to lift more, push it harder and go heavier and there have been times where my form hasn't been good. And you know what happened?

Yep, I hurt my lower back and it put me out of the game for more than six months. I was in so much pain every day at work when I had to stand around with clients and it was so sore that I had to take a lot of pain killers. I couldn't just sit down and watch my clients and there weren't any other options.

That was probably one of the most depressing times in my life because I couldn't exercise properly, I was in a world of hurt every day and it was all because I decided to show off to my own ego and lift with poor technique.

That is going to be a constant reminder for the rest of my life to just take it easy, check my ego at the door and just tortoise my way every single week. What's the point in trying to be the hare when the only person you're competing against is yourself?

BONUS TIP: HOW TO STAY MOTIVATED

What do you do once you reach your fitness goal? You've lost your target 10, 20 or 30kg, now what? Set yourself a new goal.

Find something that is going to keep you motivated to exercise and eat well day by day, whether that's a health goal or something more competitive.

At the start of this book we looked at goal-setting and having a long-term vision because it gives you a reason to keep going.

Some days you might be too tired and not want to come in to the gym. Some days you will be busy at work or at home and you will make an excuse not to exercise. Maybe you miss a day here and there and that's just life.

But when those days start adding up, it's easy to lose track, lose motivation and say, "Fuck it, life's just too busy at the moment."

That's the reason you see guys fail after a few months or a year, that's the reason they go back to what they used to look and feel like – it's because they didn't have that long-term goal or that long-term vision to motivate them to come into the gym.

It doesn't have to be anything special either.

I want to live until I'm 120. That's just my goal. But I don't want to be a brittle and frail 120-year-old. I want to be healthy and energetic, and in order to do that I need to make sure day by day I'm exercising eating the right food and doing the things that are going to get me there.

Do I do the right things every day? No.

Are there some days I don't exercise or still eat shitty food? Yep.

But having that vision reminds me to get back on track after a day or two. It's that motivating factor to keep me going.

Now, what's going to keep you motivated?

ACTION STEPS

1. Download the workout templates that I've provided for you in the resource section.
2. Pick the days you can realistically exercise on and block out those times on your calendar.
3. Pick some NEAT activities you can add into your day to burn more calories.
4. Buy yourself a foam roller to help improve your mobility and flexibility.

PART THREE

LIFESTYLE

"Progress is not achieved by luck or
accident, but by working on yourself daily"
- Epictetus -

Why am I talking about your lifestyle in a weight loss book? Why is stress, sleep and your environment so important? It's because these things play a much bigger part in your life than exercise. You sleep for more than six hours a day, you're around people all the time and you're working almost every day.

The majority of these experiences will determine your actions, what you do and the choices you make. If you can have a better management of your lifestyle and can control some of the outcomes, it will mean fat loss is going to become so much easier.

So far you've read about the diet, exercise, food and meal prep, and it's all pretty straightforward. But that's not how life plays out. There are factors like work, friends, family weekends and everything else that come up. You must learn how to manage them as well as possible.

This is coming from a guy who's a personal trainer, who's single and who has a pretty flexible life, so what I'm writing about is from my past experiences when I used to have a job and also from the experiences and struggles that my clients come to me with and that I've helped them overcome.

Most of my clients are white-collar workers who start very early in the morning and work until the wee hours of the night, sometimes 24 hours straight (lawyer clients).

They've had a lot of struggles to overcome and they still fight them continually, but here are some things that seemed to have worked so far.

9
STRESS

Stress is something we experience every day at work, in traffic and even when we're exercising. Doing exercise puts a stress on your body, but this is a good type of stress.

One thing I neglected over the years is managing my stress. I just thought it was going to be there and I had no control over it.

I used to (and still do occasionally) blow up at the simplest things. I would get angry, start yelling and just behave like a complete douchebag. It's only been the last 18 months that I've started to become much more of a calmer person and started slowing down a bit.

We all have our own ways of unwinding from stress but for many this comes in the form of drinking alcohol, watching TV or something that's really not great for your body.

Instead, you want to be able to practice a few stress-relieving methods that have been shown time and time again to work and that are more positive on your body.

MEDITATION

I'm not a woo-woo hippy guy and I'm not expecting you to be either.

When I first heard about meditation I thought it was silly. Then some of my friends told me they did it and I still laughed.

But I found myself hearing more and more about it. You know when you hear something enough you start to wonder if you should do it? Well, that was me and I thought I might as well try.

The first time I tried meditation it was horrible. In fact, the next ten times I tried meditation it was horrible. My mind was racing in a million directions, whereas I thought everything was meant to be calm.

I gave up and decided it wasn't for me. But a few weeks later I was talking to a close friend who meditated every day. I explained to him that I gave up because I couldn't turn the voices off inside of my head. "You're doing it wrong then," he said.

You see, you're not supposed to try to "turn the voices off" you're just supposed to be able to step back and watch what's going on in your head. He suggested using an app to help me, and for the next two weeks I did it every day.

I was expecting a payoff like you would see if you exercise and eat right. I was looking for some kind of like "A-ha" moment. But after 14 days there wasn't one. But I kept doing it daily because even though I didn't see any instant results, I found myself becoming less stressed and less anxious during the day.

I didn't snap at people as much and things that used to get me really angry didn't have the same effect.

So, I stuck with it and I've been a lot calmer and more focused since implementing meditation in my life. If I skip it for a couple of days now I really notice it. If you're a type A, go-getting person who lives a pretty high-stress life then you need to do some sort of meditation every day.

It could just be a two-minute breathing practice where you just stop what you're doing and concentrate on your breathing, watching yourself inhale and exhale, not trying to slow it down or speed it up, but just watching and go from there.

Being able to de-stress is going to help your body recover from exercise quicker and, more importantly, help you live longer. Living with high amounts of bad stress in your life is going to kill you and if you're not handling that stress well or you "unwind" with things that hurt your body then you're going to die sooner.

Scary thoughts, right? Here are a few suggestions for meditation.

HEADSPACE

This is the app I used to get me into the habit of meditating daily. You can download it for free and the man who walks you through the meditation has the most calming voice, just reminding you to come back to your breathing.

THREE-MINUTE MEDITATION

The second thing you can do is pick a three-minute spot in your day where you just focus on your breathing. Just put the timer on your phone, sit in a chair and focus on breathing in and out.

I know you're busy and don't have a lot of time but three minutes a day is manageable. Think about it this way; for the three to ten minutes you invest every day into managing your stress could help you live years longer, which gives you the time you've invested back and then some.

Seems like a pretty good trade-off, eh?

WHAT NOT TO DO

DON'T EXPECT A MIRACLE TO HAPPEN OVERNIGHT

The results aren't going to be instant and may not be as noticeable as you hope. But there are going to be subtle changes that you will notice over the weeks and months.

You may realise that you don't get angry in traffic as much or when the cashier is extremely slow. You may spot that you're not in that much of a rush and you just watch the world go by. But it's not all going to be sunshine and rainbows forever where you are permanently chilled out for the rest of your life either.

DON'T TRY ANYTHING FANCY

Start by just sitting in a chair – either at home or in your office – somewhere you can't be distracted. You can sit on the floor, but you don't have to try and fold yourself over and sit in a specific position like some people suggest.

Sure you can try it later, but in the early stages just focus on managing your stress and making it as easy as possible. The more resistance there is, the less likely you are to do it.

MOVEMENT

Humans are designed to move. When we move, we feel good. One of the best stress relievers is exercise.

Sometimes it's training with weights, sometimes it's hitting the boxing bag, sometimes it's just putting on some music and going for a walk around the park to chill at the end of the day.

Once you get up and start moving your body, you're going to feel that stress slowly melt away.

TALK TO SOMEONE

I'll be honest; I struggle with this one a fair bit. Guys don't really talk about their feelings as much as they should and that can be a major problem.

If you keep stuff locked up in your head, then you're going to go mental. Your mind can be your best friend and it can be your worst enemy.

Find a mate who you can talk to who's not going to bust your balls or call you a wimp but will listen to you. Alternatively, find someone who specialises in these types of things.

Just find someone you can talk to.

JOURNAL

If you don't want to talk to someone else, use a journal to note down all of your thoughts on paper.

Just getting those thoughts out of your head can help to relieve the stress. Write it out, scrunch up the paper and throw it in the bin so you don't have to worry about that shit again.

Whenever you're pissed off at the world just let it all out. It's a cool little mind trick, but it works.

> ☑ **TIP:** You can download an example of how to journal in the resource section.

FLOAT TANK

Having struggled to meditate for 15 minutes, there was no way I thought I could do a float tank. Finding out that you are there in a pitch-blank tank for an hour just letting your thoughts run wild seemed a little crazy.

But my coach urged me to give it a go (actually, he challenged me by saying I wouldn't be able to do it and I wanted to prove him wrong). After that first hour I felt so relaxed and fresh, it was amazing.

You are laying in water and epsom salts, so you're giving your muscles a bit of a relaxing massage while you lay down. It just feels great.

I only do it once a month because this is a bit more time-consuming, but it's very beneficial and you should try it.

ACTION STEPS

1. Download the meditation apps Headspace or Oak
2. Pick a time every day that you can dedicate towards trying meditation for three to ten minutes.
3. Choose an area where you won't be disturbed and either sit in a chair or on the ground.
4. Dedicate the next 14 days to doing this every single day (even on the weekends).
5. Find a friend or buy a journal to help you can get all of those crazy thoughts out of your head.

10
SLEEP

Sleep is one of the biggest factors in life that people seem to neglect. We see it more as a burden than anything else and that makes sense because we're all busy and there's so much to do.

If you sleep more, then you can't hang out with your friends as much on the weekend, or finish off that extra work you need to do that's due the following morning, right?

After a long day's work, it can be hard to come home and just switch off and go to bed. You want to unwind and chill out, so you decide to watch some TV, grab a bite to eat, check social media and the next thing you know it's midnight. Then you go to bed, but you can't seem to shut your mind off. You toss and turn and look over at the clock and you've only got two more hours until you have to get up and do it all over again.

A lack of sleep can be a huge detriment to your health. It has been shown to decrease lifespan, increase the risk of certain diseases, and it stops your body from recovering, which means you won't gain muscle as easy.

It also lowers testosterone production, increases hunger cravings and a whole lot more. When you neglect your sleep, you are killing your body and your brain.

Just because you have coffee in your life it doesn't mean that's the answer either. Most people when they're tired during the day will have a coffee to boost them up and when that coffee starts wearing off, they'll have another one.

Soon you're three to four coffees down and you think you're doing great because it's getting you through the day. But that isn't the whole story.

REDUCE THE COFFEE

Drinking three or more cups of coffee a day, especially if you're having them in the afternoon, is going to interfere with your sleep because caffeine hangs around in your body for a long time.

The average cup of regular coffee has about 80-120mg in it and it takes about eight hours for your body to metabolise half of that.

If you drink one coffee at 8am, you will still have 60mg in your system at 4pm. That means if you have four coffees during the day and your last one is at 4pm, you will still have caffeine running through your body at midnight, disrupting your sleep.

This leads to a vicious cycle of drinking lots of coffee every day just to keep you awake and alert, but also stops you from falling asleep.

You don't need to stop drinking coffee altogether, but you need to know when to stop having it during the day to get a better night's sleep.

First off, stop all caffeine consumption by 2pm. This will give your body enough to time to clear out most of the caffeine. Those who metabolise slower might have to stop earlier and switch to a green tea.

You'll know you're a slow metaboliser of coffee if you find yourself having a hard time sleeping if you have some after midday or if you feel absolutely wired after a large coffee or two cups.

If you still feel like you need something after 2pm then have some green tea or have a super dark piece of chocolate (85 per cent or more).

Another problem when you drink too much coffee is that your body can adapt to it and then you're going to need more and more to feel that same effect.

This is where coffee cycling can come in handy. There are a few ways to do coffee cycling.

WEEKLY CYCLING

Pick a few days during the week when you have coffee and some when you don't. You can play around with it to find how it suits you best. Maybe go one day on and one day off or three days on followed by three off. Perhaps you'll only drink coffee on weekdays and have the weekends off.

I usually drink my coffee as a pre-workout and stick to just one a day. Sometimes I might sneak in a second, but anything more than two and I'm paying for it. I will do this every day Monday to Saturday and then give my body a break on Sunday.

If I feel beat up and my body needs to recover, instead of the weights I'll just a light cardio day and I will skip the coffee so I'm not adding any extra stress on my body.

MONTHLY CYCLING

Once a month do one week with no coffee or any other caffeine source at all. If you like the habit of drinking coffee, like I do, you can swap your coffee for a decaf and just push through.

If you find going days without coffee isn't going to be realistic then I suggest you start small. If you drink five or six cups a day, give yourself a limit to only drinking five cups a day for the next two weeks.

Once you accomplish that, then cut it down to four cups for the next two weeks and so on until you feel like you could do a full day without coffee and see how you feel.

Because caffeine is a drug, you're going to have withdrawal symptoms and most likely these will come in the form of headaches, brain fog and morning moodiness.

This is going to be tough, so you could do half decaf, half coffee while slowly cutting back.

BEDTIME ROUTINE

Remember how when you were younger your parents used to make you get ready for bed? You would have a shower, brush your teeth, get in your pyjamas, have a drink of water and then lie down in bed while they read you a story as you slowly drifted off to sleep. Half the time they would probably only be one or two pages in and – bam! – you were out for the count.

Yet as we got older we grew out of that habit. Now we get home from work and watch TV, scroll through Facebook on our phones and then just expect to be able to fall asleep when we want to.

The problem is that because we have grown out of a bedtime routine, our body doesn't actually realise it needs to be preparing for sleep.

You need to create a routine you can follow every night before going to sleep to help your body start relaxing and winding down before you head hits the pillow.

Start getting your body ready for bed 60 minutes beforehand and ensure your phone and TV are off 30 minutes before sleep.

Create a set of relaxing steps that are going to help you unwind that doesn't include social media and watching TV.

Here's what my bedtime routine looks like.

TIME	WEIGHT
19:00	Stop all work
19:10	Warm shower
19:20	Take a scoop of magnesium with water
19:30	Finish on social media and turn phone on airplane mode
19:35	Write in my journal
19:45	Foam rolling or stretch while listening to an audiobook
20:00	Sleep

Yes, I go to bed pretty early because I need 7.5-8 hours of sleep so that I'm up and ready to rock and roll between 3.30-4am.

There are a few key things in my bedtime routine that help my body relax and get me feeling drowsy.

1. **Magnesium:** This helps your body and muscles start to relax and it's best to take this about 30 minutes before bed.
2. **Airplane mode:** It's easy to check your phone "just one more time" in case someone needs you and then get sucked into emails and Facebook and the next thing you know you've been on it for two more hours. Turn your phone on airplane mode until the morning. You will survive and Facebook will still be there.
3. **Journaling:** Being able to get your thoughts out of your head and onto paper will help clear your mind and stop you thinking about everything that has happened. If it was a crappy day, write negative stuff on paper scrunch it up and throw it away. I actually journal on my computer using an app called Evernote.

4. **Audiobook:** I'm tired at the end of the day and don't feel like reading, so I'll pop in an audiobook and have someone read to me instead. Usually, I'll either listen to an autobiography (right now I'm listening to one on Benjamin Franklin biography) or I'll listen to a fiction book.

   If you're going to read a book, make sure it's not going to stimulate your brain and keep you up all night.

5. **Stretching:** My muscles are already relaxed from the magnesium and now I'm helping undo all of the bad postures from the past day by doing some foam rolling and stretching. This is a great way to give your body a bit of love at the end of the day.

After doing these five things, I've got nothing left. I'll usually crawl into bed, put the sleep timer on my audiobook for ten minutes and I'm done.

Creating a relaxing routine for each night will work wonders.

SLEEP HYGIENE

Poor sleep hygiene can be another reason you're not getting enough sleep. If you've got a messy room, a dirty bed, you're sleeping in random clothing, it's hot or your room is lit up like Las Vegas then you're causing havoc to your body.

Your room needs to be like a dark cave-like sanctuary if you want to get the best rest possible.

This goes back to our ancestral days. When the sun went down we didn't have all of these lights shining on our eyes; we would either be sprawling out under the stars or going into our dark cave, which would have been pitch black, and gone to bed.

Now we have computer lights, phones, street lamps, and house lights shining on us all the time and this external light actually stops your body from producing melatonin, which is a chemical that is released when the body should be getting ready for sleep.

ELIMINATING EXTERNAL LIGHT

Your TV screens, your phone, street lamps, the Sun and basically everything else emits "blue light", which compared to other light sends out a higher amount of energy.

When this light hits your eyes, your brain responds by sending signals through your body to say "it's daytime". That's why you will notice an increase in energy and alertness when you go out into the sunshine during the day, because it is such a powerful blue light producer.

But because all the lights in your house and on your devices also emit blue light, your body is still getting signals saying it's daytime when it's not. This stops your body from producing melatonin and means you're not going to be able to sleep as easily.

More and more studies are showing how much light has an effect on your body when it comes to sleep and also when it comes to increasing your energy and focus during the day.

Now realistically you're not going to turn off all of your screens throughout the evening and just sit in candlelight. But you should minimise the level of blue light that your body is exposed to. Here are some steps you can take:

F.LUX

This is a free app you can download to your computer. It changes your screen's temperature at night to produce less blue light. You can get it at https://justgetflux.com.

IRIS

This is another app like F.Lux but for those who like to geek out a bit more. Iris allows you to go a bit more techy and change the screen temperature yourself or adjust it for a specific task you're doing. For example, as I write this book my computer is on the reading setting, which makes my screen black and white.

NIGHT SHIFT MODE ON SMARTPHONES

You can enable the night shift mode function on your phone, which automatically filters the blue light from your screen as it gets darker and darker at night. Both iPhone and Android phones have this feature. Google for 'night shift' on iPhones and 'night mode' for Android for instructions on how to set it for your phone.

BLUE-BLOCKING SCREEN PROTECTORS

These are screen protectors that you can put on your phone to block out the blue light if you don't have an app to do it.

BLUE-BLOCKING GLASSES

These glasses have an orange tint and you can wear them in the evenings or at night to block out the blue light from external sources including street lamps.

I wear mine at the gym from 6pm while I'm still training clients because the downlighting produces a lot of blue light.

How trendy you want to look will determine the cost of the glasses. I go out and socialise on weekends and also don't want to look like a speed dealer at the gym, so I use an awesome brand called Swannies. They're stylish, you can wear them anywhere and they work like a charm.

This brand was created from a fellow Aussie named James Swanwick, who now sells them all over the world. They also sell night masks and supplements to help you get a better night's rest.

> ☑ TIP: Find out how you can get a discount on the glasses by going to the resource section.

If you're only going to wear them around the house and aren't too concerned with how you look, then you can buy a cheap $10 pair on eBay that will do the same job.

The earlier you put on blue-blocking glasses and use the apps on your screens, the better your melatonin production will be and the better sleep you will get.

Two hours prior to bed is a good time to start using them. You will start to notice yourself getting tired earlier and be able to fall asleep that much quicker.

HAVING PAJAMAS

Do you have sets of pyjamas that you wear to bed at night? Our bodies love routine and if you include putting on a certain set of clothing at bedtime, you send yourself messages that it will soon be time to go to sleep.

You may notice that your energy levels change when you wear certain outfits. When you put on your gym kit, you'll get an energy boost as you mentally prepare for your workout.

And when you get dressed for work, you start to feel more professional and get your head in the zone.

You should also have clothes you wear to bed to signal that it's the end of the day, that there's no more work and it's time to start chilling out. I will not do any extra work once I put on my pyjamas; otherwise it's defeating the purpose.

Then, when it's finally time to go to sleep, you can either wear your pyjamas or sleep in the nude. Sleeping nude helps with cooling your body down since you're not restricted by clothing.

CLEANING YOUR ROOM

A cluttered room signifies a cluttered mind, they say. For a long time, I lived that way – working from my computer at a desk in my room with stuff everywhere.

There would be notepads, sticky notes, client programs and just piles of "stuff" around because I always had to reference something or take notes. I embraced the chaos of having "stuff".

But the problem with having my office in my room meant I felt like I couldn't relax properly at night.

One of the reasons was because it reminded me of things I have to do. I would want to come home from training clients ready to crash, but would see the papers and lists and think about all the different things that needed to be done and could not relax.

I have now made it a habit to clean my room and clear my desk once a day. At 4.15pm – before I go back to the gym to see my evening clients – I take five minutes to tidy. I put all of the crap away, pick up any clothes off the floor and have it looking schmicko.

This little habit helps clear my mind and when I come home at night, I don't get overwhelmed because my room is tidy and it feels like I have a clear mind too.

If you're someone who has a messy room or also have a desk in your room, make sure you set yourself a little goal at the end of each day just clear it all away. Even if that means opening a drawer and just throwing it all in.

If you can't see it, you can forget about it until the morning and get your body in a relaxing state.

HAVE A CLEAN BED

Not being cluttered applies to your bed, too. Don't have clothes, millions of pillows and your work gear thrown over it. The bed should be for two things – sleeping and sex.

It is not for late-night work, not an area to dump work books and clothes, and not a kitchen table to eat food.

Make your bed every morning, keep it tidy and clean, and make sure you keep it your "sacred sanctuary".

COOL AS A CUCUMBER

Growing up in North Queensland, the temperature never really dropped that low and I was always sweating. But I never had a problem with sleep because we would turn on the aircon or the ceiling fans at night to cool the room down.

We tend to sleep best when our body is at a cool temperature. You want your room to be about 16 Celsius (60 Fahrenheit).

Some people may need it a few degrees cooler or warmer. I like my room just a smidge warmer because it's already cold enough in Sydney for me.

Have a fan in your room or the aircon set to keep that temperature constant. There is nothing worse than not being able to sleep and waking up in a pool of sweat at night.

MORNING SUN

Our body has two clocks that it runs off, internal and external. You don't need a watch or phone to tell our body what time it is because we have a natural inclination on how to do that.

Have you ever told yourself that you're going to wake up at a certain time and your body seems to somehow wake you up within about 15 minutes of that time?

I find that if I want to wake at a certain time, my body will wake me up earlier as if it doesn't want me to be late. The reason your body is able to do this is because of your external clock.

The energy we receive from the Sun and the Earth help to dictate our 24-hour cycle. We want our bodies to be in sync with it, so we know when to go to sleep and when to wake up.

To align yourself with the Earth's 24-hour cycle, you need to focus on getting sunlight on your body – more specifically at two specific times of the day.

The first time should be early in the morning when the Sun starts to rise. And the earlier you expose yourself to sunlight, the easier it's going to be for your body to "sync up".

Have you ever felt really tired in the morning, gone to a local coffee shop, sat out the front on the veranda in the sunshine and it's like a wave of energy hits you?

Some of it's probably from that coffee you just drank, but most of it is from the Sun because of the powerful light it emits and how your body is receiving that light. It's basically like the Sun is saying: "Hey it's day-time, time to move your ass."

The other time you need to get sunlight is between 11am and 2pm. This is the peak time for vitamin D absorption. There are only certain times that you can get vitamin D from the Sun and it is important that you get it every day.

Getting your midday dose shouldn't be too much trouble if you get a lunch break. Get yourself outside, breathe in the fresh air and get about ten to 15 minutes every day at lunch.

The amount of time you need in the Sun is going to differ for each person. A good app to use is D minder, which will determine where you are in the world, when the best time to get vitamin D is and for how long you should spend in the sunlight. It's free to download.

When you're in the Sun, make sure you're not wearing sunglasses either. Your eyes need to be able to take in the light, so try and expose yourself as much as possible. Also ensure you're not being blocked by any windows as they will stop your body from absorbing the natural vitamin D given out.

GROUNDING

This is also going to sound a bit woo-woo but bear with me here. I also used to think this was some BS thing until I did it for myself when I travelled to the US last year.

The Earth gives off a specific frequency and energy and there are ways to "tune in" to that frequency. Grounding is when you walk barefoot on the ground and receive that frequency.

If you wear shoes all day, then you're not allowing your body to ground and align with the frequencies the Earth is sending out.

Go for a barefoot walk on some grass (walking on concrete or asphalt won't do the same thing). You need to be on land that hasn't been tampered with, so walking in a park barefoot or some soil in your backyard is a good thing to try. And make sure you aren't wearing shoes in your house.

The next time you travel to a different time zone and you don't want to have jet lag, once you've checked in to your hotel go outside for some sunlight and walk barefoot on some grass. You'll notice your body is able to adapt quickly to the new time zone.

You will have seen that I have given you a lot of information and advice on sleep. This is because it is such a crucial part of our lives and if you can master sleep, everything else becomes a lot easier.

ACTION STEPS

1. Clean your room.
2. Clear your bed.
3. Block out the blue light.
4. Create a bedtime ritual.
5. Get some pyjamas.
6. Make your room pitch black.
7. Be as cool as a cucumber.
8. Get out in the sunlight as early as possible.

11
FRIENDS, FAMILY AND WEEKENDS

The weekend is not a special occasion. Everyone uses it as an excuse to slack off from their diet or exercise. But let's be real here, the weekend isn't anything special. It comes around 52 times a year, just like every other part of the week does.

If you decide to slack off just because "it's the weekend" then you're letting all of the hard work you've put in during the week come undone.

A stall in fat loss usually happens because of the amount of food and alcohol that is consumed from Friday to Sunday.

You go out for drinks after work on Friday and then get some greasy food. You wake up Saturday morning and go out to get a big breakfast, then you go out for lunch, meet up with friends for Saturday afternoon drinks or someone's birthday and then you have another greasy meal for dinner, maybe two.

Sunday morning rolls around and it's bacon and eggs for the ultimate pick me up (healthy fats, right?). Maybe there's also a Sunday sesh down at the pub. The next thing you know you've slammed down over 10,000 calories in a weekend all coming from fatty food and alcohol. And then you wonder why you can't lose weight.

But don't worry, you don't need to stop drinking alcohol altogether, you just need to learn how to manage it.

This is where intermittent fasting becomes such a powerful tool, because you're still able to go out with your friends to have a few beers but not worry about the extra fat gain that comes with it.

Go back to the diet part of the book and look at how much food you've determined that you need to eat during the week in order to lose weight.

Let's say you need 2,400 calories a day. Across seven days that amounts to 16,800 calories.

In terms of weight loss, it doesn't really matter how many of those calories you eat on each individual day. What matters is that you do not exceed the total for the week.

If you eat 2,400 calories each day Monday to Thursday but then 3,000+ on Friday, Saturday and Sunday, then you've just undone your hard work.

But if you know you're going out on a Saturday night then consume less during the week to compensate for your weekend.

If you know that on Friday night you plan on going out with your mates and you plan to have ten or so drinks, you can account for that ahead of time. The average beer is 160 calories so that equals around 1,600 extra calories that night.

So, here's what you could do: From Thursday night until Friday night you do a full 24-hour fast. This means that on Friday night you could have a small 800 calorie meal (lean protein and vegetables) and also ten drinks, which would let you hit 2,400 calories for the day.

Another way you could do this is to eat 300 fewer calories every weekday. So, from Monday to Friday, you eat 2,000 to 2,100 calories and when Friday night rolls around you've "saved" yourself about 1,500 calories to play with for a good time.

This is not an exact science and won't always play out that easy, but when you start to think about it like this it's so much easier to live a fun lifestyle with your mates and enjoy a few drinks while maintaining your diet.

If you go over the number of planned calories on a Friday or Saturday night out, you can do a full 24-hour fast the next day. This way you've got the chance to keep your calories low and maintain that calorie deficit that you put yourself in during the week.

Why doesn't this work for most people on diets? It's because they eat the exact same amount of calories every day and a small hiccup here and there or one big hiccup can bring it all crashing down and they don't know how to manage it. Or they haven't created a big enough deficit during the week in order to minimise the effect.

So many of my clients go out and drink with their friends during the weekend and still get lean by using this approach. Speaking of which, Aaron, one of my online clients, has carved out six-pack and lean physique and has kept it even while travelling through Europe and partying every night.

I'm not saying I condone this approach, I'm just showing you that it can be done.

What you've probably realised is how calorifically high alcohol is and it's a bitch. This is one of the reasons I don't drink (and also because I'd much rather eat my food and be full). I also know that I'm going to be losing weight every week, rather than stressing out about going out on a Saturday night and trying to figure out how many calories I need to "save" during the week.

My advice would be to quit drinking. It's not good for you, makes you feel like shit and makes weight loss so much harder.

Now I know you probably won't listen to that advice, so let's try another approach. Let's work on just lowering the amount of alcohol you drink.

If you usually drink 12 to 15 drinks each week then we want to work on a habit-based approach to drop that down.

For the next two weeks, set yourself a goal to have no more than 12 drinks a week. After the two weeks is up and you successfully didn't go over the 12-drink limit, you would then drop it to 11 a week for another two weeks, and then ten drinks and so on.

This way you're slowly reducing the amount of alcohol you're drinking every two weeks and you're not really noticing. But over time those small changes will wind up making a huge difference. In two months from now you will have gone from having 12 drinks every week down to eight.

You're saving yourself about 600 calories, saving yourself about $32 and – more importantly – saving your internal organs and having a better quality of life.

This brings us back to the thinking behind "cheat days". People often ask when they can have a cheat day or if it's OK to have one if you aren't following an intermittent fasting diet.

It's very hard to "get away" with having a cheat day, because most people don't tend to be in a big enough calorie deficit.

Another problem with cheat days is that people feel like they can just eat and drink whatever they want all day for one day and that it's a good thing to do it because they "need it".

Why do you need a cheat day? Do you really need to eat as much food and drink as much alcohol in such a short period of time, make yourself feel like shit and then repeat that process once a week because you feel so deprived of certain foods?

Cheat days lead you to feel guilty and throw you backwards when it comes to your dieting.

If you have a big appetite and have a cheat day, then you could end up eating more than 7,000 to 8,000 calories in that one day.

Instead of thinking about cheat days, why not just add the things you like into your diet and follow the 90/10 plan?

Calculate how much you need to eat every day to achieve your goals and decide whether that ten per cent is going to be one small thing each day or more of a treat meal on the weekend when you go out with friends for a few drinks.

And don't call it cheat. What are you cheating on? This should be a treat meal, and you know what "treat" means right? It means only on occasion.

It doesn't mean that every single day you're filling your gob with foods that are bad just because they fit into your calories for the day.

I'm going to say it again; I'm here to help your body thrive, not just survive and every time you fill your body with crap, you're not doing it justice.

BONUS TIP: HOW TO TELL FRIENDS YOU'RE NOT EATING

It can be a bit weird if you're invited out for breakfast or to a family event and you're the only person at the table not eating. It's happened to me plenty of times.

But people will only think it's odd if you make a big deal out of it or tell them about what you're doing.

Instead, you can just tell people you don't like having breakfast in the morning, that you don't feel hungry or that you don't feel the best right now and you'll just have a coffee.

It will be hard to resist the temptation of food, but you will get used to it.

I recently went on a boat cruise with some friends for a charity event and there was dinner included. Since I had just started my fast, I wasn't going to eat anything else for the day.

When we got on the boat there were more than 200 boxes of pizza. There was literally enough that everyone could have had one each.

But I didn't even bat an eyelid over it. Yes, it smelled good but, after practising intermittent fasting for so long, the thought of eating any of it didn't cross my mind.

This won't happen for you straight away, but those small wins when you start off will soon add up.

You don't have to discuss your intermittent fasting with your friends, because most of the time they will tell you about how you should try some other type of diet because of this benefit or that, and then you're going to get into a conversation you didn't want to have in the first place.

ACTION STEPS

1. Brainstorm how you can change your "cheat meals" into treat meals.
2. If you're going out on a weekend or to a special event, make sure you plan out your week to eat less every day so you're in a calorie deficit.

12
BUILDING HABITS IN THE MORNING

Habits take time to build and they're a bitch to break. Some of the habits you've built up over your life have served you well, but others not so much. But that's the great thing about habits – they can be broken and built up over time.

Think about the things you do in the morning when you get out of bed: Drink some coffee, have a shower, read the newspaper and grab a bagel on the way to work.

When you become aware of a habit, good or bad, you're able to change it. And the best time to do this is in the morning.

When you wake up is when you have the most willpower and you are pretty much at your best. Nothing has got in your way yet and the slate is clean – making this the perfect time to start a new habit.

Pick one habit you want to change and make the alteration first thing in the morning. Let's use exercise as an example.

You've been slack with your exercise lately and you know you need to get back into it. You have good intentions, pack your kit the night before and tell yourself that you'll go straight to the gym after work. But something comes up.

The boss needs you to stay back, you remember you have to run to the store to pick something up or you just feel too drained after work.

We've all been there. And when we try again and the same thing happens, we decide to give up.

Instead of planning to go to the gym in the afternoon, go in the morning before the rest of the world gets at you. Some of my most successful clients have made the habit of coming to see me in the morning because they know it's the only time can really go, and this is the time where there are no distractions.

So whether that be hitting the weights or doing a cardio session, do it in the morning. The sooner you get it out of your way, the sooner the rest of the day is yours to do what you want. Studies have also shown the benefits of working out in the morning to improve sleep, productivity and focus at work, and your mood.

HABITS TAKE TIME TO BUILD

We have good and bad habits and they didn't just form overnight. They take time to build up. But in the same way you've subconsciously built up bad habits, you will also have good ones.

A good rule of thumb for forming a new habit is between 20 and 60 days. That's a big swing in variation but it really depends on the person.

Set yourself a good habit of morning exercise that is aligned with your goals for the next 12 weeks to keep that habit ingrained.

COMMON PITFALLS

Many will say they aren't a "morning person". That's probably because they stay up until 11pm or midnight watching TV and feel tired in the morning, right? If you live like that then it's expected that you wouldn't be a morning person.

You need to think about what time you go to bed and how that dictates if you're a morning person.

If you go to sleep earlier, you will wake up earlier and that will give you a chance to go to the gym. And you don't need to miss out on your shows because you can watch your Netflix on your phone or tablet while you're doing your cardio in the morning, remember?

THINKING YOU'RE BETTER THAN THE AVERAGE PERSON

Others might say: "It might take normal people 20 to 60 days to form a habit, but I'm different. I can do it in two weeks."

This type of thinking has left a lot of people in trouble in the past and it will probably cause problems for you too.

We like to think we're not the average person and we're smarter, better, faster, etc. but in reality, that's not true. We are all very similar in our habits. If you want to make sure that new habit becomes ingrained, then ensure you stick at it for 12 weeks. Even if you are that special person who can form a habit it two weeks, you will be doing yourself an even bigger favour.

CREATING TOO MANY HABITS

Don't try and change everything at once. Taking on too much will lead to failure.

From a standing start, people will say: "I'm going to cut out all unhealthy food, I'm going to meal prep every morning before my workout, I'm going to ride to work, I'm going to quit drinking and this all starts tomorrow."

Be honest, how many times do you think that all-in approach has worked? Instead, focus on creating small wins first. While you are going to cut out trigger foods and alcohol for your first month that doesn't mean you're going to keep them away forever.

Exercising every morning is a great starting place for fitness and meal prepping once a week is a great for nutrition.

This isn't a Get Ripped Quick book; this is about changing your health and your fitness for life.

BONUS TIP: AVOIDING FALLING OUT OF GOOD HABITS

You are going to have all of the best intentions in the world to eat healthier, exercise more, reduce the amount of alcohol you drink and pretty much do a "full reset" of your health and fitness. But here's the truth – you're lining yourself up to fail if you try and do everything at once.

If you try and cut out all unhealthy food, go to the gym seven times a week and avoid drinking altogether, you might be able to last one week or maybe even a month or three, but you're going to fall off the bandwagon eventually.

Think about the other diets you've tried or the times you've tried to implement a new habit and it didn't work. My goal is to set you up for long-term success.

The point of this book wasn't to get you shredded in six weeks; it was to get you to transform your lifestyle step-by-step so you're able to maintain the changes you make for the rest of your life.

In order to do that you need to start small. Set goals that you're able to stick to before moving on to something else. Tell yourself that you're only going to eat four pieces of chocolate a week instead of five pieces or have ten bottles of beer instead of 12.

If you haven't been to the gym in months or years, then a goal of going two or three times a week is more realistic than seven times a week.

Remember, the only person you're racing is you.

"The chains of habit are too weak to be felt until they're too strong to be broken."

Consistent action that you can stick to day-to-day is better than doing a shit load of action for a short amount of time and then going back to your old habits.

Let me give you an example. A while ago I was trying to fix my sleep. I was coming home after work and sitting on social media for an hour, then getting in bed and texting my clients for the next day, and I was wondering why I felt run down in the mornings. I knew what the issue was, so I decided to make a change.

But instead of making a small habit-based change, I thought I was better than that because "I'm a trainer and I know best." I decided that as soon as I would come home, there would be no social media, no nothing – just a shower and straight to bed.

This worked for two weeks and then it all came crashing down.

I was missing out on talking to friends and one night I thought I would just jump on for a few seconds and I got sucked in. I woke up the next day and felt terrible and thought to myself, "OK, I'm not going to do that again."

The next night I did the exact same thing and the night after that. I had tried to completely overhaul a bad habit without trying to minimise it slowly first.

I had to swallow my pride and realise that I need to make small steps like everyone else.

So, I decided to limit myself to 40 minutes of social media for two weeks. That was easy at first and every night I kept telling myself I can do less I can do less, but I was ignoring that ego and giving myself "permission" to stick to my rules.

Two weeks after that I reduced it down to 30 minutes a night and I noticed that my sleep got a lot better. I was now able to socialise after work, but also still have time to unwind and chill before I go to bed.

My limit is still 30 minutes and I don't plan on going any less than that because it's enough to do some browsing and chat with friends without it interfering with my sleep.

Keep in mind that you are going to have to change your habits gradually with micro-commitments, but all of those micro-commitments over time will completely change your bad habit.

ACTION STEPS

1. Decide to stick to the intermittent fasting diet for the next 60 days to build in a new habit.
2. Pick one day a week you can meal prep for the next six weeks.
3. Decide how long you can exercise every day and put it in your calendar.

13
A WORD OF WARNING

It's day one and you're excited, you've decided that you're going to start intermittent fasting this week and you're ready to go. You wake up and you're feeling good. This is the start of something new; you know this time it is going to work.

This time is different.

Since you're skipping breakfast, you find yourself with a little bit more of free time, so you just hang around at home before work. You grab your meals that you prepared yesterday out of the fridge and you're on your way to work.

So far, so good.

Morning hunger starts to kick in and your stomach growls, but you knew this would happen because you read about it in this book, so you decide to drink some sparkling water and 20 minutes later the hunger pangs are gone.

You're banging away on your keyboard getting lots of work done, not even worrying about food. Before you know it, it's 12pm and you've just completed your first 16-hour fast.

"Wow, easier than I thought. This is a piece of cake," you say.

You have your first meal and realise how much better the food tastes. Why does this meal taste so good? You realise it's because this is the longest your body has gone without food.

You repeat this for the next five days and it goes off without a hitch. Sunday rolls around again and you prepare your meals for the following week. You're on a high because you've just knocked out your first week and you're feeling great. But then it's hot on the Sunday night and you can't sleep properly. Your alarm goes off and you have to peel yourself out of bed, splash some cold water on your face to wake you up and go to the coffee pot downstairs.

You sip on the coffee while reading the paper and then you realise, "Shit, I've got to hand in the project today." You rush to work and get there before everyone else to get the work done. Suddenly it's 9.30am and you're starving.

You need to focus, you need to get this work done, but you're tired and you can't concentrate. You need that little bit of sugar to drive you through to lunch, maybe a Snickers bar?

Warning: This is temptation calling out.

Do you really need the Snickers bar? Do you really want to throw in the towel after just seven days of intermittent fasting?

You're having a fight in your head back and forth and you don't know what to do. Your good intentions get the best of you and you decide to make yourself another black coffee instead of buying a Snickers bar.

The coffee helps to push you on for another 90 minutes and it's now 11am. Again, you start to feel the dip in energy and your stomach is now really growling.

A co-worker brings back a box of doughnuts and is offering them around to everyone.

You're watching him come closer and closer and you want that dough-nut. You're craving that sugar and there's this little voice at the back of your head telling you, "It's OK. Have the doughnut. You're tired. You can have one. It'll give you a boost."

You're ready to give in and you're just waiting for him to come over to you. You can taste it!

But he doesn't come to you.

Why not? Then you remember that last week you told everyone in the office that you're on a new diet and you need their help to not offer you any temptations.

Thank God they listened.

You get distracted by your work again and soon it's midday. You remember that you forgot the lunch you prepared at home and you're starving. You need something quick because you have to get back to finish this project.

Toasted sandwich? Pork roll? Thai food? Then a thought pops into your head. You've got frozen veggies in the freezer at work and you can pick up a quarter piece of roast chicken from around the corner.

You have prepared!

You eat your lunch and you're feeling good about yourself. A few hours ago, you were on the brink of caving in and now you're still on track.

You beat temptation.

That sort of temptation is going to show up all the time when you're trying to achieve a goal. You need to become aware when this happens and have a plan to beat it.

There are going to be days when you forget to pack a healthy lunch, when you're offered unhealthy food or when you have a crappy sleep and you want to throw in the towel.

That's temptation and that's when it's the most important time for you to push through and persevere. But since you know temptation is going to show up, you can put things in place to make sure you don't fall off track.

You have learned about preparing meals, keeping frozen vegetables at work, keeping hydrated and putting little things in place that help keep you on track. There's a reason those things are so important.

When you prepare ahead of time, you're setting yourself up to win when temptation comes knocking. When you prepare you will overcome those tough times.

When you prepare, you win. You beat temptation. You knock that bitch down for another day.

But don't get cocky. It will show up again and again. It's not going to stop and it's going to appear in different ways.

Maybe next week it's the temptation to skip meal prep on Sunday because all your friends want to go out for breakfast. Maybe it's having the cake at lunch because it's your colleague's birthday. The temptation will show up, but you can beat it.

What choice are you going to make when that comes up? Prepare ahead and you will win.

CLOSING THOUGHTS

What a journey! You've now got all the information you need to live a fitter, healthier lifestyle and it's now up to you to put that information into action. You don't have to change everything in one go, like I said, start slowly and make a few small changes at a time before going all in.

This isn't an overnight thing. Ditch The Diet means following an intermittent fasting lifestyle, exercising regularly and having the flexibility to suit it around your lifestyle – but this is a process. It's going to take time and you're going to make mistakes, but this book is here to help you get back on track, and so am I.

I want you to join my Facebook group where you can keep in touch, ask questions, share your wins and be surrounded by like-minded people following this approach.

I also want you to send me your before and after transformation photos having followed what you've learned in this book. There is nothing I love more than seeing transformations made by people following my advice. Send your results and pictures to: tyson@tysonbrown.com.au – I promise I'll respond.

By the way, you can also connect with me on social media:

Facebook: www.facebook.com/tysonthetrainer
Instagram: www.instagram.com/tysonthetrainerr
Snapchat: @tysonbpt
Twitter: @tysonthetrainer

HOW TO TRAIN WITH TYSON

If you're ready to make the changes in your life that you have now seen are possible through this book then I'd love to help you out. You can kick that stubborn fat to the curb once and for all and live a much healthier life by having a customised nutrition and workout plan that's tailored around your busy life and your goals. Let me take care of the nitty gritty details and create an easy-to-follow guide that tells you exactly what you need to do every day in order to get the body you desire.

If you'd like to apply for online coaching, visit this webpage and fill out the form to request a free coaching call:
http://www.tysonbrown.com.au/online-coaching/

Once you apply, I'll be in touch to set up our call.

I'd also love to connect with you on social media, so make sure to join the private Facebook group by going here:
https://www.facebook.com/groups/transformingwithtyson/

Carmel Cox "I have seen amazing results, especially in weight loss and muscle definition. Tyson is passionate about fitness and diet, bringing a charged enthusiasm and energy whenever we talk."

Max Young " Tyson helped me kickstart my fitness journey. Together we built the foundations of what has now, undoubtedly, become a lifelong habit. His holistic approach towards fitness ensured guaranteed results – through coaching me about my thoughts and attitude, providing a culture of friendship, accountability and responsibility, high quality training and a systemic approach to health and fitness that takes into account so many important factors like sleep, nutrition, recovery, mobility and longevity. Since then I've lost 10kgs of fat, I'm training consistently without the need for "motivation". I'm building muscle, increasing my strength and overall sense of satisfaction in life. Through training with Tyson, I was able to realise that I am so much more capable that I think I am, physically, mentally and emotionally – and that has made all the difference in my life."

GLOSSARY

High intensity interval training (HIIT)
Short bursts of high-intensity (or max-intensity) exercise followed by a brief low-intensity activity, repeatedly, until too exhausted to continue.

Low intensity steady state (LISS)
Light cardio about 50 to 60 per cent of your maximum heart rate at a consistent pace, usually for long durations.

Non-exercise activity thermogenesis (NEAT)
Non-exercise related activity that you do during the day such as walking your dog, riding your bike to the shop or sitting down.

Intermittent fasting
An umbrella term for various diets that cycle between a period of fasting and non-fasting during a defined period

Autophagy
Consumption of the body's own tissue as a metabolic process occurring in starvation and certain diseases.

Brain derived neurotrophic factor (BDNF)
Helping to support the survival of existing neurons, and encourage the growth and differentiation of new neurons and synapses.

Insulin sensitivity
How sensitive your body is to insulin.

RESOURCES

All downloads mentioned in the book – such as the 30-day reset, workout template and recipes – can be downloaded from my website: www.tysonbown.com/book-bonus

Here is a list of the products I recommend in the book.

Supplements

- **Fish oil (great for heart health, brain health and joint protection)**
  http://bit.ly/iherbfishoil

- **Magnesium (good for muscle recovery and relaxing before bed)**
  http://bit.ly/magnesiummuscle

- **Swannies (blue light blocking glasses to help you sleep)**
  http://bit.ly/swanniesglasses

- **Protein (perfect for meeting your daily protein needs)**
  http://bit.ly/iherbproteinpowder

- **Creatine (helps build additional strength)**
  http://bit.ly/iherbcreatine

- **Vitamin D**
  http://bit.ly/iherbvitamind

- **Sleep mask (blocks out all external light)**
  http://bit.ly/sleepmastermask

Digital products

- **MyFitnessPal (a great app to track your food)**
  https://www.myfitnesspal.com

- **Audible (to listen to a book instead of reading it)**
  https:// www.audible.com

- **D minder (the best time to get sunlight based on your location)**
  iPhone: http://bit.ly/dminderiphone
  Android: http://bit.ly/dminderandroid

- **Kindle app reader (take your books anywhere you go)**
  http://bit.ly/kindlebookapp

- **Netflix (the perfect way to take your mind off cardio)**
  https://www.netflix.com

- **Oak (a meditation app to help you relax)**
  iPhone: http://bit.ly/oakiphone

- **Headspace (another meditation app to help you relax)**
  https://www.headspace.com

F.Lux (cuts out the blue light from computer screens)
  https://justgetflux.com/

- **Iris (a more advanced version of F.Lux)**
  https://iristech.co/

- **Interval Timer (to track your HIIT workouts)**
  Android - http://bit.ly/intervaltime1
  iPhone - http://bit.ly/intervaltimer2

KEEP IN TOUCH

I hope you have enjoyed learning about how you can get in the fast lane to achieving your fitness goals and I wish you every success.

Need more help? Do you want to join me? Here's how!

- Become a member of my Facebook tribe www.facebook.com/transformingwithtyson
- Apply for online personal training – www.tysonbrown.com.au/online-coaching/
- Download my podcasts – Tyson's Fitness Tips from your podcast app

Share your success stories with me. I'd love to hear from you.

Email them to: tyson@tysonbrown.com.au

Or post on: www.facebook.com/transformingwithtyson

To your Success,

Tyson

www.ingramcontent.com/pod-product-compliance
Lightning Source LLC
Chambersburg PA
CBHW060853280326
41934CB00007B/1026